Current Concepts in Surgical Pathology of the Pancreas

Guest Editors

N. VOLKAN ADSAY, MD
OLCA BASTURK, MD

SURGICAL PATHOLOGY CLINICS

surgpath.theclinics.com

Consulting Editor
JOHN R. GOLDBLUM, MD

June 2011 • Volume 4 • Number 2

SAUNDERS an imprint of ELSEVIER, Inc.

W.B. SAUNDERS COMPANY
A Division of Elsevier Inc.

1600 John F. Kennedy Boulevard ● Suite 1800 ● Philadelphia, Pennsylvania 19103-2899

http://www.surgpath.theclinics.com

SURGICAL PATHOLOGY CLINICS Volume 4, Number 2
June 2011 ISSN 1875-9181, ISBN-13: 978-1-4557-0512-2

Editor: Joanne Husovski

Surgical Pathology Clinics (ISSN 1875-9181) is published quarterly by Elsevier Inc., 360 Park Avenue South, New York, NY 10010. Months of issue are March, June, September, and December. Business and Editorial Office: Elsevier Inc., 1600 John F. Kennedy Blvd., Ste. 1800, Philadelphia, PA 19103-2899. Accounting and Circulation Offices: Elsevier Inc., 3251 Riverport Lane, Maryland Heights, MO 63043. Periodicals postage paid at New York, NY and at additional mailing offices. Subscription prices are $170.00 per year (US individuals), $199.00 per year (US institutions), $84.00 per year (US students/residents), $213.00 per year (Canadian individuals), $225.00 per year (Canadian Institutions), $213.00 per year (foreign individuals), $225.00 per year (foreign institutions), and $104.00 per year (international & Canadian students/residents). Foreign air speed delivery is included in all *Clinics'* subscription prices. All prices are subject to change without notice. **POSTMASTER:** Send address changes to *Surgical Pathology Clinics*, Elsevier, 3251 Riverport Lane, Maryland Heights, MO 63043. Customer Service: 1-800-654-2452 (US). From outside the United States, call 1-314-447-8871. Fax: 1-314-447-8029. E-mail: JournalsCustomerServiceusa@elsevier.com (for print support) and JournalsOnlineSupport-usa@elsevier.com (for online support).

Reprints. For copies of 100 or more, of articles in this publication, please contact the Commercial Reprints Department, Elsevier Inc., 360 Park Avenue South, New York, NY 10010-1710. Tel. (212) 633-3812; Fax: (212) 462-1935; E-mail: reprints@elsevier.com.

Printed in the United States of America.

Contributors

CONSULTING EDITOR

JOHN R. GOLDBLUM, MD
Chairman, Department of Anatomic Pathology;
Professor of Pathology, Cleveland Clinics,
Lerner College of Medicine, Cleveland Clinic,
Cleveland, Ohio

GUEST EDITORS

N. VOLKAN ADSAY, MD
Professor and Vice-Chair; Director of Anatomic
Pathology, Department of Pathology and
Laboratory Medicine, Emory University,
Atlanta, Georgia

OLCA BASTURK, MD
Department of Pathology, Memorial
Sloan-Kettering Cancer Center,
New York, New York

AUTHORS

N. VOLKAN ADSAY, MD
Professor and Vice-Chair; Director of Anatomic
Pathology, Department of Pathology and
Laboratory Medicine, Emory University,
Atlanta, Georgia

OLCA BASTURK, MD
Department of Pathology, Memorial
Sloan-Kettering Cancer Center, New York,
New York

GIUSEPPE BOGINA, MD
Department of Pathology, Ospedale Sacro
Cuore Don Calabria, Verona, Italy

LAURA BORTESI, MD
Department of Pathology, Ospedale Sacro
Cuore Don Calabria, Verona, Italy

PAOLA CASTELLI, MD
Department of Pathology, Ospedale Sacro
Cuore Don Calabria, Verona, Italy

TOBY C. CORNISH, MD, PhD
Clinical Fellow, GI and Liver Pathology,
Department of Pathology, The Sol Goldman
Pancreatic Cancer Research Center, The
Johns Hopkins Medical Institutions, The Johns
Hopkins Hospital, Baltimore, Maryland

ALTON B. FARRIS III, MD
Department of Pathology and Laboratory
Medicine, Emory University Hospital,
Emory University, Atlanta, Georgia

RALPH H. HRUBAN, MD
Professor of Pathology and Oncology,
Department of Pathology, The Sol Goldman
Pancreatic Cancer Research Center,
The Johns Hopkins Medical Institutions,
The Johns Hopkins Hospital, Baltimore,
Maryland

DAVID S. KLIMSTRA, MD
Chief, Surgical Pathology Service, Memorial
Sloan-Kettering Cancer Center, New York,
New York

ALYSSA M. KRASINSKAS, MD
Associate Professor, Department of
Pathology, Presbyterian Hospital,
University of Pittsburgh Medical Center,
Pittsburgh, Pennsylvania

TOSHIO MOROHOSHI, MD
First Department of Pathology, Showa
University School of Medicine, Tokyo, Japan

NOBUYUKI OHIKE, MD
First Department of Pathology, Showa
University School of Medicine, Tokyo,
Japan

ANNA PESCI, MD
Department of Pathology, Ospedale Sacro
Cuore Don Calabria, Verona, Italy

MICHELLE REID, MBBS
Assistant Professor of Pathology, Department
of Pathology, Emory University Hospital,
Atlanta, Georgia

LAURA H. TANG, MD, PhD
Assistant Attending Pathologist, Department
of Pathology, Memorial Sloan-Kettering
Cancer Center, New York, New York

BENOÎT TERRIS, MD, PhD
Professor, Department of Pathology, Paris
Descartes University, Cochin Hospital, Paris,
France

GIUSEPPE ZAMBONI, MD
Department of Pathology, Ospedale Sacro
Cuore Don Calabria; Department of Pathology,
University of Verona, Verona, Italy

Contents

Pancreatic ductal adenocarcinoma (PDAC) and its variants comprise between 80% and 90% of all tumors of the exocrine pancreas. Because of its silent course, late clinical manifestation, and rapid growth, it is considered a silent killer. Only 10% to 15% of cases are resectable and the 5-year survival rate remains lower than 5%. The differential diagnosis between PDAC and chronic pancreatitis is a challenge for pathologists. This article provides a guide for pathologic evaluation of PDAC specimens with the macroscopic and microscopic features of common PDAC and its variants and discusses the differential diagnosis and morphologic and immuno-phenotypical prognostic parameters.

Pancreatic intraepithelial neoplasias (PanINs) are microscopic lesions of the pancreas. Traditionally viewed as a benign metaplasia of small ducts, evidence suggests that PanINs are neoplastic and that some PanINs progress to invasive ductal adenocarcinoma. The primary diagnostic challenge is distinguishing PanINs from other lesions, including invasive ductal adenocarcinoma, intraductal papillary mucinous neoplasm, and cancerization of benign ducts. PanINs are the most common of the pancreatic cancer precursor lesions, yet they remain poorly understood and are so small that they are almost clinically undetectable. Further study is required to define the role of PanINs in the carcinogenesis and early detection of pancreatic cancer.

This article presents the clinicopathologic characteristics and differential features of pancreatic mucinous tumors. These tumors, which correspond to the most frequent cystic neoplasms, are encountered with increasing frequency. They comprise the mucinous cystic neoplasms and the intraductal papillary mucinous neoplasms. These tumors are known to progress from dysplasia to invasive carcinoma. Thus, it appears important to distinguish them from other cystic neoplasms and non-neoplastic cysts.

Cystic lesions of nonmucinous type can arise within the pancreas or can develop from adjacent structures and appear to involve the pancreas. In addition, some typically solid masses can become cystic or can present as cystic lesions. Nonmucinous cysts can be neoplastic, inflammatory, reactive, or congenital. The vast majority of neoplastic nonmucinous cysts are benign. Because of the difficulty in determining the neoplastic potential of a pancreatic cyst preoperatively, many non-neoplastic cysts are resected. This article reviews the surgical pathology of nonmucinous cysts.

This review describes the clinicopathologic characteristics, differential diagnosis, and biologic behavior of exocrine pancreatic tumors of predominantly nonductal differentiation: acinar cell carcinoma, pancreatoblastoma, and solid-pseudopapillary neoplasm. Patients usually present with a well-demarcated, large, soft, solitary mass with expansile, rather than infiltrative, growth pattern. Cystic change is common. Histologically, the tumors usually reveal at least a focal solid, cellular appearance composed of uniform, monomorphic epithelial cells. However, each type has characteristic clinicopathological features. The immunohistochemical labeling profile of pancreatoblastoma parallels the multiple lines of differentiation. These tumors are capable of producing metastases; however, their behavior is different among the types and even in the same type. Therefore, establishment of a grading system that can predict the outcome would be helpful.

Pancreatic neuroendocrine tumors (Pan-NETs) are the second most common epithelial neoplasm of the pancreas after ductal adenocarcinoma. They can be clinically defined as functional, nonfunctional, and hereditary. This review addresses typical and atypical pathologic features of Pan-NETs, with a focus on practical issues involved in differential diagnosis, immunohistochemical workup, intraoperative frozen section interpretation, sources of diagnostic errors, and classification. The diagnosis of a Pan-NET requires analysis of all available clinical and radiographic information and pathologic characteristics of the tumor, and it is crucial to understand the clinical impact of the pathologic interpretation.

The pancreas is versatile in the diversity of disorders that it can exhibit. In this article, characteristics of disorders such as chronic, autoimmune, eosinophilic, hereditary, and infectious pancreatitis are described. With regard to autoimmune pancreatitis, the role of clinical evaluation, histologic examination, and IgG4 immunohistochemistry is discussed. The role of pancreatitis in the pathogenesis of diabetes is also mentioned. Some implications of pancreatitis are highlighted, including the neoplastic predisposition caused by inflammatory lesions of the pancreas. The goal of this article is to convey an appreciation of these disorders because their recognition can benefit patients tremendously, as inflammatory lesions of the pancreas can be mass-forming, giving rise to pseudotumors, and leading to surgical resection that may otherwise be unnecessary.

Pancreatic cytopathology plays a critical role in the management of patients with cystic and solid pancreatic masses. The frequency of pancreatic fine-needle aspiration continues to increase and general surgical pathologists and cytopathologists need to be aware of the most commonly encountered entities as well as the pitfalls associated with gastrointestinal tract contaminants in endoscopic ultrasound-guided fine-needle aspiration. This article focuses on the most commonly encountered pancreatic lesions and the importance of correlation of cytologic features with clinical, radiologic, and ancillary studies for accurate diagnosis.

Surgical Pathology Clinics

THE CLINICS ARE NOW AVAILABLE ONLINE!

Access your subscription at:
www.theclinics.com

The Pancreas: From Sweetbread to A Diagnostic Challenge

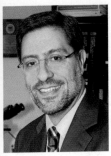 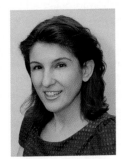

N. Volkan Adsay, MD   Olca Basturk, MD

Guest Editors

The saga of pancreas began with the ancient Greeks at the coastal bays of the Aegean Sea, now a part of modern Turkey, where the term pancreas was coined (the Greek root of the word is based on the cow pancreas being a gourmet food, "sweetbread"). Its first anatomic dissection was performed (without any understanding of its associations), and the first speculations on its nature and significance (it was believed to be a mere cushion for the vessels lying behind it) had been made. It may be an interesting coincidence for the readers to note that both guest editors of this issue were originally from the Aegean region, too. Much has been learned about this enigmatic organ since the days of Galen, but at the same time, undoubtedly much remains to be unraveled. We hope that we were true to our ancestors and that this issue reflects a compact review on the pathology of the pancreas as we currently understand it.

For surgical pathologists, the pancreas has been a challenging specimen. In the past, this was mostly due to a lack of familiarity due to the rarity of the specimen. Until recently, pancreato-duodenectomy was rarely performed because it was seen as a high-mortality operation that is to be avoided at all cost. When Whipple published his series in 1941, the overall mortality rate was 30%. For decades, this figure had remained fairly high, which fueled the reluctance to perform this much-feared operation. However, the improvements in surgical techniques and perioperative care in the past two decades have dramatically reduced the mortality rate of the "Whipple" operation to less than 2% in experienced hands. Now, a modified version of "Whipple" operation is performed routinely not only in major medical centers but in many smaller community hospitals as well.

Meanwhile, from the 1980s onward, the advancements of imaging technology have made the pancreas infinitely more accessible and thus pancreatic pathology, including "incidentalomas," in particular the cystic lesions, has begun to come to clinical attention routinely during daily practice. Consequently, CT-guided core biopsies and EUS-guided fine-needle aspiration biopsies have become a part of initial work-up and brought a whole new horizon to pancreas pathology.

All of these have led to an increase in the number of the pancreas specimens pathologists encounter on a daily basis and, in turn, advanced our knowledge of this organ. New entities were described, and the pathogenesis, morphology, and biology of the entities already known were studied in more detail.

Therefore, we believe that it is very timely to have a comprehensive and practical coverage of the current concepts, diagnostic criteria, differential diagnosis, and clinical/biologic behavior of main pathologic conditions of the pancreas. The issue starts with by far the most common and most important malignancy in the pancreas: ductal adenocarcinoma, followed by precursor lesions (PanINs). We would like to emphasize here that it is largely underappreciated that pancreatic ductal adenocarcinoma is the fourth leading cause of cancer deaths in the United States and in many

Surgical Pathology 4 (2011) ix–x
doi:10.1016/j.path.2011.05.001
1875-9181/11/$ – see front matter

other developed countries. Since 2004, more Americans died of pancreas cancer than of prostate and it appears that the number of deaths from this cancer type will surpass that of the breast within the next couple of years. Ductal adenocarcinoma is also one of the most common sources of carcinoma of unknown primary. Mucinous and nonmucinous cystic lesions are discussed separately because they constitute two different categories as mucinous cysts have well-established malignant potential, and those that are nonmucinous such as serous cystadenomas have no malignant potential. The former is a very important category also for cancer researchers because it is a distinct and more indolent pathway of carcinogenesis in the pancreas and thus offers an invaluable group to analyze the mechanisms of cancer formation. Other exocrine pancreatic tumors, namely acinar cell carcinoma, pancreatoblastoma, and solid-pseudopapillary neoplasm, are covered together within the same article due to the overlap in their morphological and genetic features. Another article focuses on pancreatic neuroendocrine tumors, a much debated subject in pancreas pathology. Both the terminology and the approach to the diagnosis of these tumors have changed tremendously in the past few years. Another article outlines inflammatory lesions and pseudotumors because recognition of their key diagnostic features is important for proper clinical management. Finally, an article on cytology is added as the frequency of pancreatic fine-needle aspiration continues to increase and general surgical pathologists and cytopathologists need to be aware of the most commonly encountered entities as well as the pitfalls. Each article is detailed in a diagnostic sense and is punctuated by key features, differential diagnosis, and potential pitfalls boxes summarizing the most important aspects of specific entities. A large number of high-quality color photomicrographs illustrate the most relevant features discussed in the text.

We are indebted to the authors, who have contributed superb reviews of the topic, incorporating their own personal experience into a thorough review of the current concepts and controversies. Their hard work and expertise in these challenging areas of diagnostic pathology have been invaluable in making this issue possible. We hope that this issue will serve as a useful resource to pathologists in their daily practice.

We would like to thank John Goldblum for the invitation to guest edit and acknowledge Joanne Husovski for her patience, organizational skills, and patronage during the completion of this project. We are also indebted to our colleagues, trainees, teachers, and mentors for their countless contributions to our knowledge. Finally our special thanks to the Adsay, Basturk, and Cheng families. We are extremely fortunate to have tremendously supportive families that allow and motivate us to pursue these endeavors.

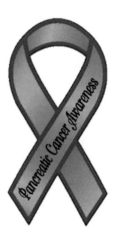

N. Volkan Adsay, MD
Department of Pathology and Laboratory Medicine
Emory University
1364 Clifton Road NE, Room H-180B
Atlanta, GA 30322, USA

Olca Basturk, MD
Department of Pathology
Memorial Sloan-Kettering Cancer Center
1275 York Avenue
New York, NY 10065, USA

E-mail addresses:
volkan.adsay@emory.edu (N.V. Adsay)
basturko@mskcc.org (O. Basturk)

DUCTAL ADENOCARCINOMA OF THE PANCREAS

Laura Bortesi, MD[a], Anna Pesci, MD[a],
Giuseppe Bogina, MD[a], Paola Castelli, MD[a],
Giuseppe Zamboni, MD[a,b,*]

KEYWORDS

- Pancreas • Pancreatic cancer • Pancreatic neoplasms • Pathology

ABSTRACT

Pancreatic ductal adenocarcinoma (PDAC) and its variants comprise between 80% and 90% of all tumors of the exocrine pancreas. Because of its silent course, late clinical manifestation, and rapid growth, it is considered a silent killer. Only 10% to 15% of cases are resectable and the 5-year survival rate remains lower than 5%. The differential diagnosis between PDAC and chronic pancreatitis is a challenge for pathologists. This article provides a guide for pathologic evaluation of PDAC specimens with the macroscopic and microscopic features of common PDAC and its variants and discusses the differential diagnosis and morphologic and immunophenotypical prognostic parameters.

BACKGROUND: PANCREATIC DUCTAL ADENOCARCINOMA

Pancreatic ductal adenocarcinoma (PDAC) and its variants comprise between 80% and 90% of all tumors of the exocrine pancreas, although ductal cells account for only 10% to 30% of the normal pancreatic parenchyma.[1,2] Because of its silent course, late clinical manifestation, and rapid growth, it has been considered a silent killer.[3] It represents the fourth leading cause of cancer death in the United States, among both men and women.[4] In Italy it ranks 11th and 10th among the most frequent cancers in men (2.2% of all cancers) and women (2.8% of all cancers), respectively, representing the 7th most frequent cause of cancer deaths (4.6% of all cancer deaths) among men and the 6th (6.6%) among women.[5]

Despite significant improvements in diagnostic imaging and the introduction of fine-needle aspiration (FNA) biopsy with the possibility of obtaining preoperative morphologic diagnosis, only 10% to 15% of cases are resectable and the 5-year survival rate remains lower than 5%.

With the exception of functioning endocrine tumors, characterized by a specific clinical picture, other pancreatic tumor masses manifest with

Key Points
DUCTAL ADENOCARCINOMA

1. Ductal adenocarcinoma comprises 80% to 90% of all tumors of the exocrine pancreas and is considered a silent killer.

2. It is characterized by a proliferation of infiltrating duct-like and tubular structures embedded in abundant desmoplastic stroma.

3. It is a highly invasive neoplasm with diffuse perineural and vascular infiltration.

4. The main and more challenging differential diagnosis is with chronic pancreatitis (CP).

[a] Department of Pathology, Ospedale Sacro Cuore Don Calabria, Via don Sempreboni 5, 37024 Negrar, Verona, Italy
[b] Department of Pathology, University of Verona, Ple. Scuro 10, 37134 Verona, Italy
* Corresponding author. Department of Pathology, Ospedale Sacro Cuore Don Calabria, Via don Sempreboni 5, 37024 Negrar, Verona, Italy.
E-mail address: giuseppe.zamboni@sacrocuore.it

Surgical Pathology 4 (2011) 487–521
doi:10.1016/j.path.2011.03.007
1875-9181/11/$ – see front matter © 2011 Elsevier Inc. All rights reserved.

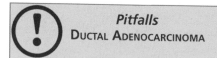

Pitfalls

DUCTAL ADENOCARCINOMA

! Differential diagnosis with CP

! Differential diagnosis with mass-forming autoimmune pancreatitis (AIP)

! Presence of cell atypia on cytologic samples in a context of inflammation

! Lack of radiologic and clinical information

either nonspecific symptoms or symptoms similar to pancreatitis. Common symptoms of PDAC are painless jaundice, epigastric pain that radiates to the back, weight loss, nausea, and pruritus. Most pancreatic cancers are diagnosed between the ages of 60 and 80 years, although sometimes they occur in younger patients (younger than age 40 years).

Although a correct diagnosis of PDAC is mandatory for planning an the appropriate therapeutic approach and establishing a prognosis, the differential diagnosis between PDAC and CP is a well-known challenge for pathologists, not only on cytology, biopsy specimens, and frozen sections but also sometimes on resected specimens. Other reasons for this difficulty are that resection specimens of pancreatic cancer are not everyday occurrences in most pathology departments and

the intriguing anatomic complexity encountered in a pancreatoduodenectomy specimen. Nevertheless, pathologists play a vital role in the team of specialists. To paraphrase the title of an article on the role of pathologists in colorectal cancer,[6] "the pathologist, the surgeon and pancreatic cancer—get it right because it matters."

This article provides a practical guide for the pathologic evaluation of resected specimens of PDAC with the macroscopic and microscopic features of common PDAC and its variants. It discusses the differential diagnosis and the most relevant morphologic and immunophenotypical prognostic parameters.

GROSS FEATURES

Ductal adenocarcinomas are firm masses with poorly defined and infiltrative borders, yellow to white in color. Hemorrhage and necrosis can be observed, particularly in larger tumors. A prevalent cystic appearance may be rarely observed as a result of massive degenerative phenomenon or secondary to the development of retention cysts. Most resected PDACs of the head of the pancreas have a mean greatest dimension of between 2.5 cm and 3.5 cm.[7] Carcinomas of the head of the pancreas usually invade the common bile duct and/or the main pancreatic duct and produce abrupt stenosis with dilatation in the upstream ductal system and fibrous atrophy of the parenchyma (**Fig. 1**). In more advanced cases, the duodenal wall and the papilla of Vater

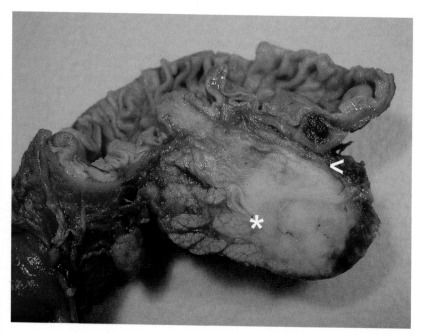

Fig. 1. Cross-section of infiltrating ductal adenocarcinoma with solid, white to yellow, sclerotic, and ill-defined mass. Common bile duct (*arrowhead*) and duct of Wirsung (*asterisk*).

can be involved. Carcinomas of body/tail are usually larger.

The macroscopic distinction of CP from PDAC may be difficult. In alcoholic CP, the scarring areas, with the exception of late stage, are inter-mixed with preserved lobular parenchyma, and calculi and extrapancreatic pseudocyst can be frequently present. Whenever present, the steno-sis of the bile duct is not abrupt but shows a tapering appearance. In paraduodenal pancreatitis, fibrotic and cystic changes are preferentially located in the region of the papilla minor and involve the duodenal wall and the groove between the duodenum and the pancreas.[8,9] In focal-type AIP, the distinction from PDAC is difficult. The absence of duct of Wirsung dilatation may be useful.[9]

The duodenopancreatectomy specimens should be examined in the fresh, unfixed state (this is less important for left-side resections). The common bile duct and the main pancreatic duct should be probed (**Fig. 2**A) and the whole specimen cut horizontally along the probes (see **Fig. 2**B). The site of the tumor should be recorded in relation to the ampulla, the pancreatic duct, and the common bile duct to exclude ampullary or terminal bile duct carcinomas. The macroscopic features that can be useful in the identification of

Fig. 2. Carcinoma in the head of the pancreas: the duct of Wirsung (*asterisk*) and the bile duct (*arrowhead*) are probed (*A*) and cut hori-zontally (*B*).

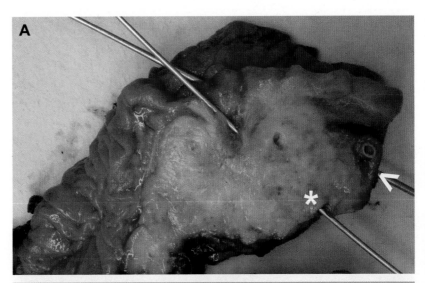

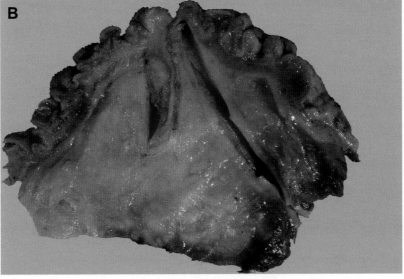

those invasive ductal carcinomas associated with preinvasive neoplasms are intraductal tumor growth, the presence of mucus in intraductal papillary mucinous neoplasms (IPMNs), and the absence of ductal connection in the mucinous cystic neoplasms (MCNs).

Completeness of resection should be assessed by gross examination and confirmed by histologic examination. Because the most frequent site of local recurrence of PDAC involves the retroperitoneal posterior bed of the pancreas, the most important tissue to study is the peripancreatic fibrous and adipose tissue that runs behind the head of the pancreas and dorsally and laterally to the superior mesenteric artery (retroperitoneal margin) (**Fig. 3**A). This area, as well as the posterior surface of the pancreas, should be inked and sectioned perpendicularly and 4 to 5 successive, numbered cassettes should be submitted for histologic examination (see **Fig. 3**B). Protocols have been published by the College of American Pathologists (http://www.cap.org/apps/docs/committees/cancer/cancer_protocols/2009/PancreasExo_09protocol.pdf), the Royal College of Pathologists (http://www.rcpath.org/resources/pdf/datasethistopathological reportingcarcinomasmay10.pdf), and many other groups.[7,10–12]

MICROSCOPIC FEATURES

Microscopically, PDAC is characterized by a proliferation of infiltrating duct-like and tubular

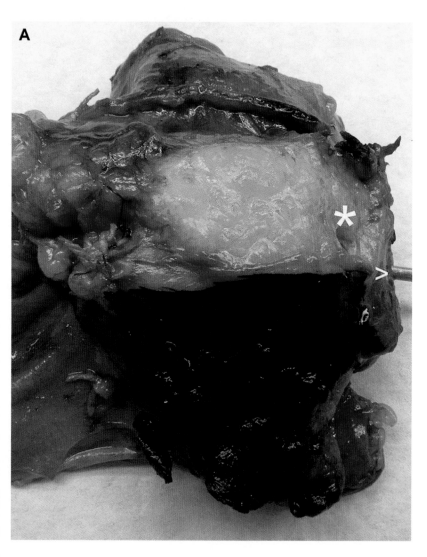

Fig. 3A. Pancreatoduodenectomy specimen. The superior mesenteric vein groove is inked in blue and the adipose tissue running dorsally and laterally to the superior mesenteric artery (retroperitoneal margin) in black. Common bile duct (*arrowhead*) and duct of Wirsung (*asterisk*).

Fig. 3B. Pancreatoduode- nectomy specimen. The inked retroperitoneal mar- gin is sectioned perpendic- ularly and the numbered cassettes submitted for his- tologic examination.

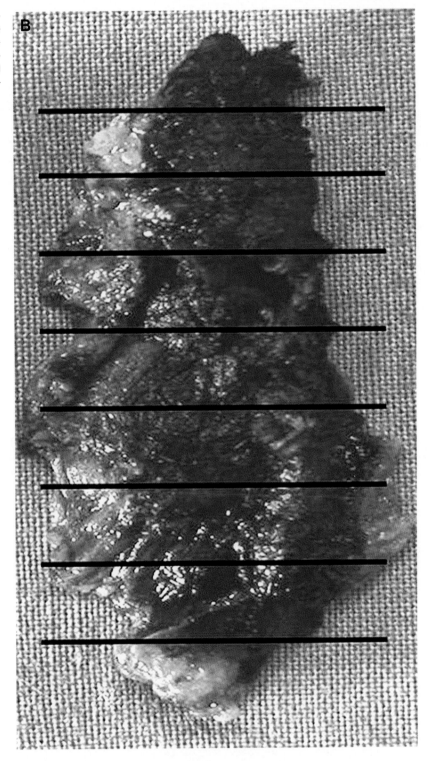

structures embedded in abundant desmoplastic stroma, which gives the macroscopic scirrhous appearance. The neoplastic tubules or glands are lined with cuboidal or cylindrical cells, frequently with large and irregular nuclei and clear cytoplasm containing a variable amount of mucin (**Fig. 4**). The degree of gland formation is proportional to the degree of differentiation and

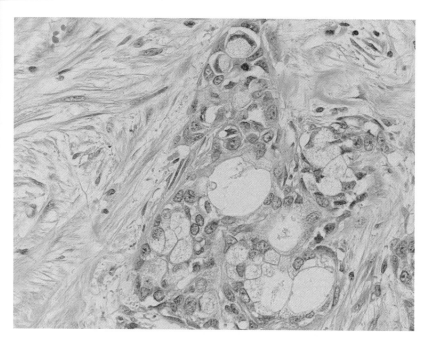

Fig. 4. Ductal invasive adenocarcinoma, characterized by well-differentiated glands surrounded by desmoplastic stroma.

can vary from well-formed glands to hardly identifiable glandular structures to solid sheets or single infiltrating neoplastic cells. The desmoplastic stromal reaction, which in most cases outnumbers the neoplastic epithelial component, is made of myofibroblast, lymphocytes, and other inflammatory cells.

At low magnification, the most striking aspect of PDAC is its invasiveness. The neoplastic glands are not restricted to the main bulk of the tumor

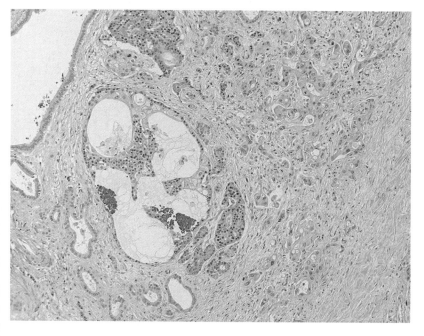

Fig. 5. Neoplastic ductuloinsular complex, showing the presence of endocrine cells associated with the ductal neoplastic cells.

Fig. 6. Haphazard distribution of neoplastic glands that lack the normal lobular pattern.

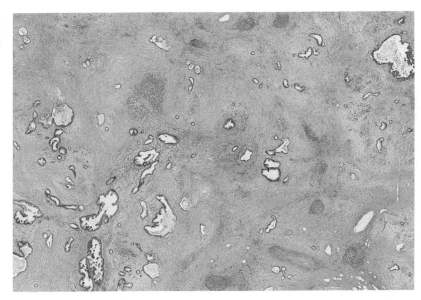

and invade the surrounding pancreatic parenchyma, both the interlobular connective septa and the epithelial exocrine and endocrine components, the vessels, the nerve trunks, and the peripancreatic adipose tissue. They can invade and grow inside the surrounding pancreatic ducts, inside the bile duct, and along the basal membrane of ampulla and duodenal epithelium. In some cases, the carcinomatous glands are associated with a non-neoplastic endocrine cell component, forming neoplastic ductuloinsular complexes (**Fig. 5**). Characteristically, the neoplastic glands are haphazardly distributed (**Fig. 6**), whereas the so-called tubular complexes that

Fig. 7. Perineural invasion.

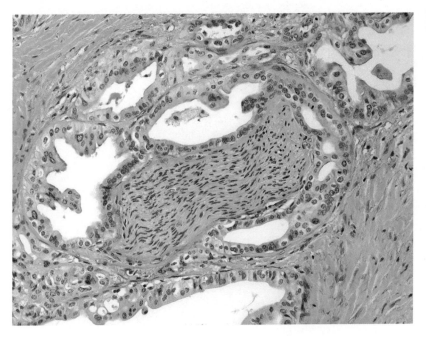

can be found in CP retain the normal lobular arrangement, with a central pancreatic duct surrounded by dilated small ductules, smoothly demarcated from the surrounding fibrotic tissue.

The presence of extrapancreatic tissue invasion is essentially diagnostic of PDAC. Perineural, vascular, and duodenal wall invasions in most cases are simple to recognize. In other cases, it can be less obvious to consider well-differentiated glands as truly invasive, such as glands close to muscular arteries, the replacement of normal endothelium of the vessels by neoplastic epithelium, or the presence of individual naked ducts in the adipose tissue.

Perineural infiltration probably represents the most typical finding in PDAC, detected in almost all cases (**Fig. 7**). Although benign pancreatic ducts can be found close to nerve trunks, they almost never invade the perineurium; only extremely rare examples have been reported.[13]

The vascular invasions, frequently found in the extrapancreatic parenchyma, usually involve the lymphatic vessels. The veins can be also involved. When the neoplastic cells invade the intima, they can replace the normal endothelium, producing a difficult-to-recognize vascular invasion (**Fig. 8A**). This lesion can mimic a pancreatic intraepithelial neoplasia (PanIN). The knowledge of its existence

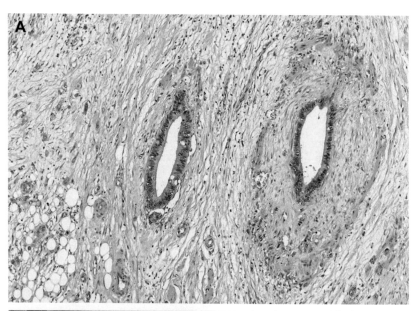

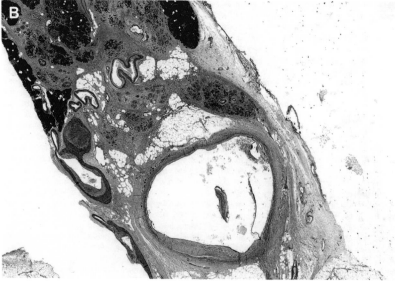

Fig. 8. Infiltrating ductal adenocarcinoma with vascular invasions, replacing the endothelial lining, with preservation (*right*) and partial destruction of the vessel wall (*center*). On the left, neoplastic single cells infiltration (*A*). Splenic vein with neoplastic intimal invasion. Double immunostaining (*B*) with smooth muscle actin (*brown*) and keratin (*red*).

and the staining for the smooth muscle and epithelial markers can facilitate its recognition (see **Fig. 8**B).

The presence of glands immediately adjacent to muscular vessels without intervening acini is highly suggestive of PDAC, because in the normal pancreas the ducts are separated from muscular vessels by the acinar parenchyma (**Fig. 9**).

The presence of naked glands touching adipocytes is almost diagnostic of carcinoma (**Fig. 10**). In pancreatic lipomatosis and CP, the glands are frequently surrounded by a rim of fibrous stroma or may be associated with some survived acinar or insular cells.

Due to obstruction of the main pancreatic duct or one of the secondary ducts by the PDAC, obstructive CP characterized with ductal dilatation, atrophy of the acinar cells, and replacement by fibrous tissue might develop.

At higher magnification, the glands and tubular structures are variably pleomorphic with variation in nuclear size of 4:1 among the cells within an individual gland. The finding of basally located, large, atypical, and hyperchromatic nuclei in a well-differentiated gland constituted by equally sized cells is diagnostic of carcinoma. The presence of mitotic figures in glands and tubular structures strongly suggests a carcinoma.[7] Well-differentiated adenocarcinomas are composed of well-defined, medium-sized glands (**Fig. 11**). The glands are frequently complete and only occasionally incomplete or with cribriform and micropapillary projections. The lining cells vary from cuboidal to columnar, with basally oriented, uniform, round to oval nuclei that have evenly dispersed chromatin. Minimal nuclear pleomorphism and rare mitosis are seen.[2,14] In moderately differentiated carcinomas, the size and shape of the glands are more heterogeneous (**Fig. 12**). Incomplete glandular lumens are common. The nuclei are more pleomorphic and hyperchromatic and the nucleoli are evident. Mitoses are common and may be atypical.[2,14] Poorly differentiated adenocarcinomas are characterized by the presence of poorly formed glands, with individual infiltrating cells, and solid areas. Necrotic foci are common. The neoplastic cells show marked nuclear pleomorphism and little mucin production (**Fig. 13**). Mitoses, including atypical mitoses, are common.

Infiltrating PDAC can be histologically graded. The grading system developed by Klöppel and colleagues (**Table 1**),[15,16] based on the degree of glandular differentiation, mucin production, nuclear atypia, and mitotic activity, has been shown to have prognostic significance. This system, based on the most undifferentiated component, might be considered complex and time consuming in everyday

Fig. 9. Infiltrating ductal adenocarcinoma with glands adjacent to a muscular vessel.

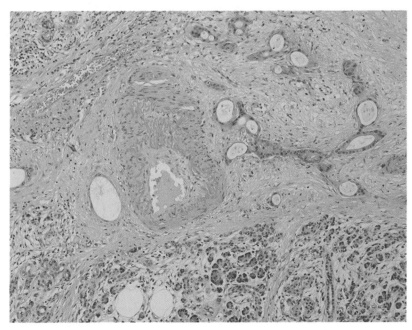

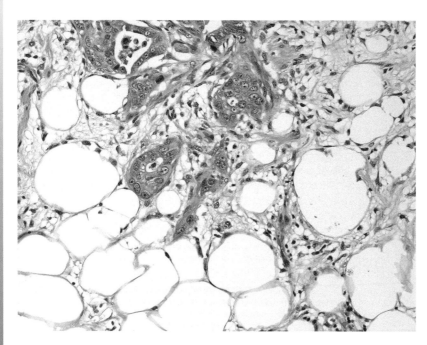

Fig. 10. Naked neoplastic glands close to the adipose tissue.

practice. A simpler and prognostically relevant grading system that parallels the Gleason grading system for prostatic carcinoma has been proposed by Adsay.[17] In this grading system, patterns (P) of infiltration are classified as follows: P1, well-defined glands with easily discernible contours; P2, fused or poorly formed glands with ill-defined contours; and P3, nonglandular patterns. A score

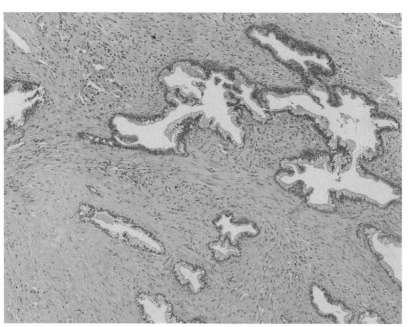

Fig. 11. Well-differentiated adenocarcinoma.

Fig. 12. Moderately differentiated adenocarcinoma.

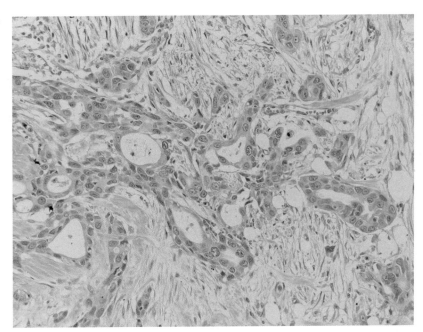

is then obtained by the summation of the predominant and the secondary patterns.

PDAC in most cases is composed of conventional glands and tubular structures. Several morphologic patterns can be observed in a pure form or, more frequently, found within a conventional adenocarcinoma. Although these patterns do not seem to have peculiar clinical and prognostic characteristics and for this reason are not included in the variants, their knowledge may help in the differential diagnosis.

A foamy gland pattern is characterized by bland, benign-appearing cells with a prominent microvesicular cytoplasm that gives a foamy appearance (**Fig. 14**). It has to be differentiated from low-grade PanIN.[18]

Fig. 13. Poorly differentiated adenocarcinoma.

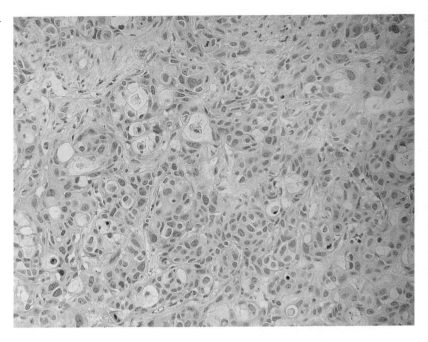

Table 1
Histologic grading of pancreatic ductal adenocarcinoma

Grade	Glandular Differentiation	Mucin Production	Mitoses (per 10 HPF)	Nuclear Features
1	Well differentiated	Intensive	≤5	Little polymorphism, polar arrangement
2	Moderately differentiated duct-like structures and tubular glands	Irregular	6–10	Moderate polymorphism
3	Poorly differentiated glands, mucoepidermoid and pleomorphic structures	Abortive	>10	Marked polymorphism and Increased size

Data from Klöppel G, Lingenthal G, von Bülow M, et al. Histologic and fine structural features of pancreatic ductal adenocarcinomas in relation to growth and prognosis. Histopathology 1985;9:841–56.

A clear cell pattern is characterized by abundant clear cell cytoplasm, resembling renal clear-cell carcinoma.[19] In cases of a prevalent solid component, the presence of mucin, immunoreactivity for pancreatic markers, and negativity for CD10 may be useful (**Fig. 15**).

A large duct pattern is characterized macroscopically by the presence of microcysts, less than 1 cm in dimension and not detectable radiologically (**Fig. 16**).[7,20] These are the 2 most important features to be considered in the differential diagnosis with an intraductal neoplasm, which has a better prognosis. At low magnification, the large duct proliferation lacks a normal lobular arrangement and may be found in abnormal locations. At higher magnification, the glands show bland appearance (**Fig. 17**).

IMMUNOHISTOCHEMISTRY

In PDAC, the tumor cells consistently express MUC1 (**Fig. 18**); like the normal intralobular small

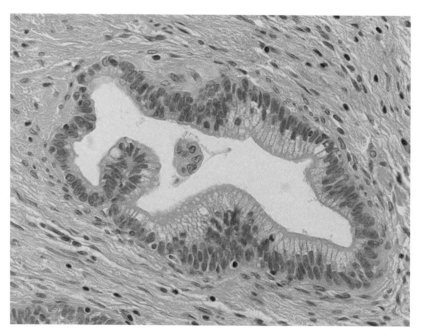

Fig. 14. Foamy gland pattern.

Fig. 15. Clear cell pattern. (*A*) Hematoxylin-eosin and (*B*) MUC1 immunoreactivity.

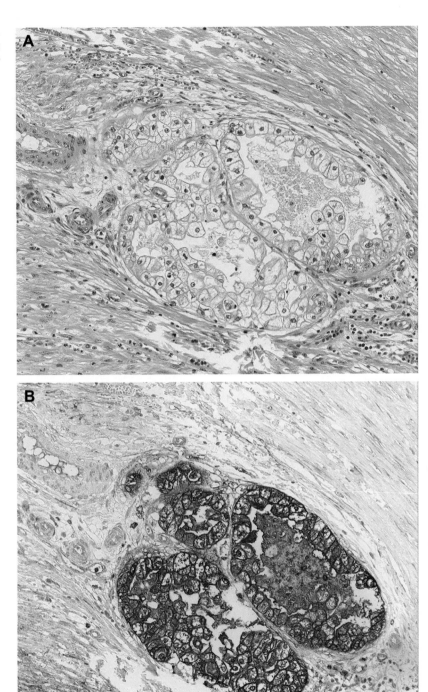

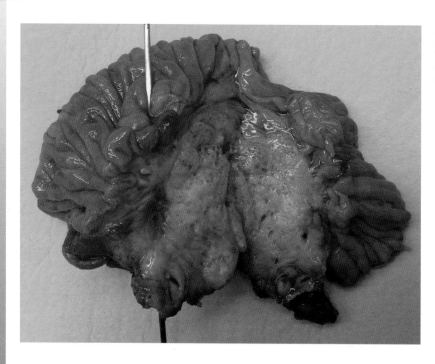

Fig. 16. Large duct pattern of adenocarcinoma. White, sclerotic mass in the head of the pancreas with multiple small cysts.

ductules, most express MUC4 and MUC5. MUC2 is expressed in a minority of cases, in which intestinal differentiation may be morphologically evident (**Fig. 19**). Other markers typically found in adenocarcinomas are the cytokeratins 7, 8, 18, 19, and occasionally 20; CA19-9; DUPAN-2 and carcinoembryonic antigen (CEA); mesothelin; CA125; and TAG-72.[7,14]

The 2 more useful markers to distinguish PDAC from the reactive glands in CP, although not

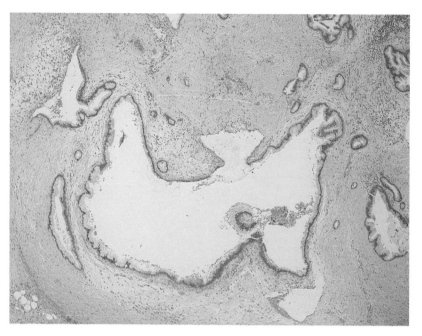

Fig. 17. Large duct pattern of adenocarcinoma with well-differentiated glands.

Fig. 18. Infiltrating ductal adenocarcinoma, immunolabeling for MUC1.

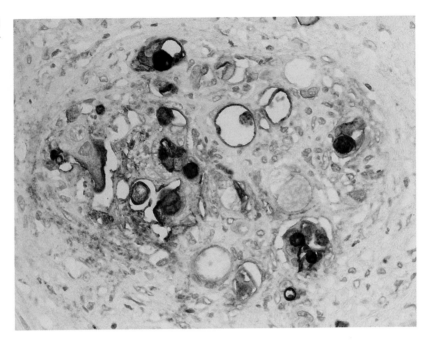

completely sensitive and specific, are the loss of Smad4/DPC4 (**Fig. 20**) and a strong positivity for p53.[7]

ADENOCARCINOMA VARIANTS

Although closely related to the conventional type, variants of PDAC are a distinct group of tumor types important to recognize because of significant clinicopathologic features, depending on the specific type. This category of tumors includes adenosquamous carcinoma, colloid carcinoma, signet ring cell carcinoma, hepatoid carcinoma, medullary carcinoma, undifferentiated carcinoma, and undifferentiated carcinoma with osteoclast-like giant cells.

Fig. 19. Infiltrating ductal adenocarcinoma with intestinal differentiation (immunoreactivity for MUC2 in goblet cells).

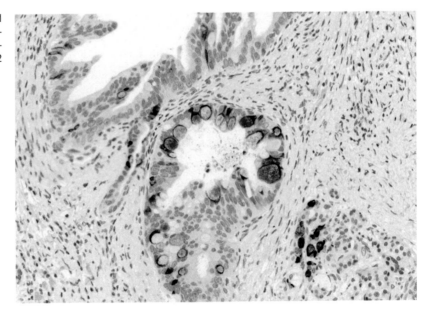

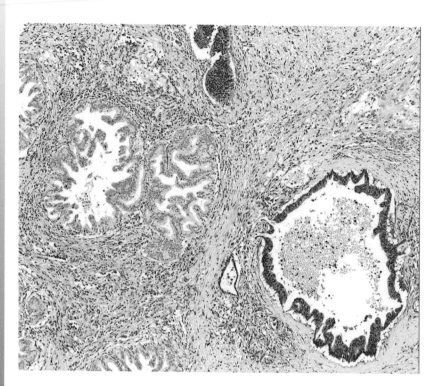

Fig. 20. Loss of DPC4 nuclear expression in the neoplastic gland (*left*); the non-neoplastic ducts maintain the nuclear immunoreactivity (*right*).

ADENOSQUAMOUS CARCINOMA

Adenosquamous carcinoma is a malignant exocrine neoplasm composed of a mixture (>30%) of 2 neoplastic components, a glandular component and a squamous cell component. The diagnosis of pure squamous carcinoma of the pancreas, a rare neoplasm, should be made only after extensive sampling of the tumor to exclude the presence of a malignant glandular component.[7,21,22] The differential diagnosis with metastatic squamous carcinoma is essentially based on clinical information. Adenosquamous carcinomas account for 1% to 4% of all pancreatic cancers.[23,24]

Macroscopically, the adenosquamous carcinomas generally are large firm masses (**Fig. 21**) and sometimes they can be cystic. It is not clear

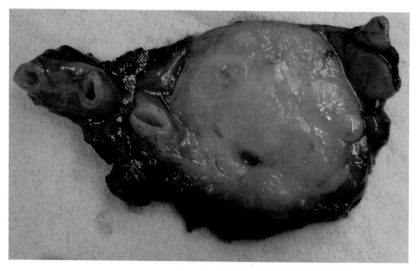

Fig. 21. Cross-section of adenosquamous carcinoma of the body of the pancreas.

whether they show a topographic prevalence.[7,25] Microscopically, the squamous component is characterized by infiltrating sheet-like arrangement of polygonal cells with distinct cellular borders, evident intracellular junctions, eosinophilic cytoplasm, and varying degrees of keratinisation. The solid nests frequently show, intermingled with the squamoid cell component, large cells with abundant clear staining cytoplasm, which may be vacuolated. These vacuolated cells show positive staining for periodic acid–Schiff (PAS)-positive diastase-resistant mucins and/or alcian blue. In some, a peripheral alcian blue and a central dot PAS positivity can be observed, creating a targetoid pattern (**Fig. 22**).

The squamous component can be intimately admixed or topographically separate to the adenocarcinomatous component within the neoplasm (**Fig. 23**A).[23]

The grading of adenosquamous carcinomas should consider 2 components: the adenocarcinoma is graded as a conventional type whereas

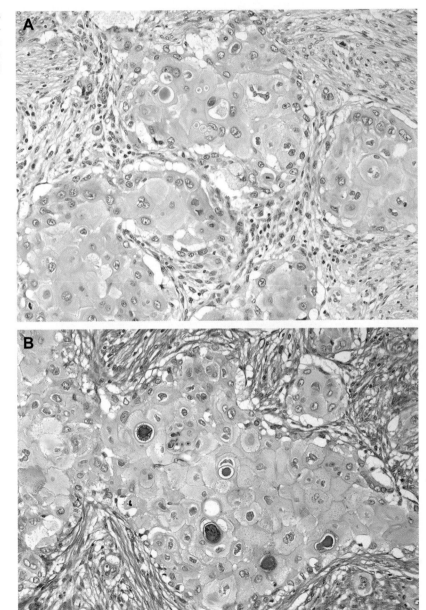

Fig. 22. Adenosquamous carcinoma with vacuolated cytoplasms with targetoid pattern. (*A*) Hematoxylin-eosin and (*B*) alcian-PAS.

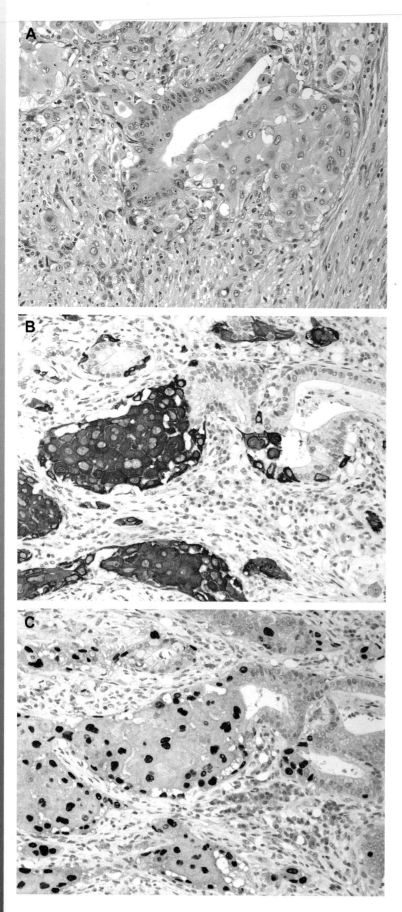

Fig. 23. Adenosquamous carcinoma with squamous and glandular component. (*A*) Hematoxylin-eosin. Immunoreactivity for keratin 5 (*B*) and p63 (*C*) in the squamous component.

the squamous component can be characterized by benign-appearing squamous elements (adenoacanthoma) or by well-differentiated or poorly differentiated squamous cell carcinoma.[7]

Metastatic adenosquamous carcinomas can present with both components or with only one (most frequently the adenocarcinomatous one).[23]

The immunohistochemical profile is similar to ductal adenocarcinoma with loss of p16, loss of Smad4/DPC4, and strong p53 expression. The squamous component often expresses CK5/6 and p63 (see **Fig. 23**B, C).[26] Both components, tubular and squamous, show MUC1 immunoreactivity. Most neoplasms have activating point mutations in codon 12 of *KRAS* gene.[21]

Adenosquamous carcinoma is an extremely aggressive neoplasm (median survival 7–11 months).[24,27,28]

COLLOID CARCINOMA

Colloid carcinoma is an infiltrating adenocarcinoma characterized by the presence of mucin-producing neoplastic cells floating in large pools of extracellular mucin. The colloid component should comprise at least 80% of the mass.[29] The epithelial cells are usually well differentiated and often present at the edges of the pools with clusters going to the center of the pools. Signet ring cells can be present.

Macroscopically, the tumor is usually well demarcated and shows a gelatinous appearance (**Fig. 24**). Microscopically, colloid carcinomas almost always arise in association with an intestinal-type IPMN (**Fig. 25**).[30,31] The finding of a colloid carcinoma in the pancreas should prompt a pathologist to search for an IPMN. It is important to differentiate benign mucin spillage often present in these neoplasms from a true invasion. Mucin spillage consists of mucus lakes without floating neoplastic cells often associated with inflammation. Perineural and lymphatic invasion is not as common as ductal adenocarcinoma.[7] The neoplastic cells express the intestinal differentiation markers, MUC2 and CDX2 (**Fig. 26**), not significantly expressed in conventional PDAC. Resected tumors have a more favorable prognosis than ductal adenocarcinoma, with a reported 5-year survival rate of 57%.[32] Pseudomyxoma peritonei can be a rare complication.

SIGNET RING CELL CARCINOMA

Signet ring cell carcinoma is a malignant neoplasm predominantly composed of infiltrating noncohesive cells with intracytoplasmic mucin, which displaces the nucleus toward the periphery, creating the signet ring cell appearance (**Fig. 27**).[33] Cells may be associated with

Fig. 24. Cross-section of colloid carcinoma of the head of the pancreas with gelatinous appearance.

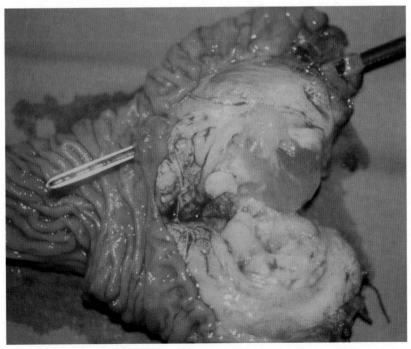

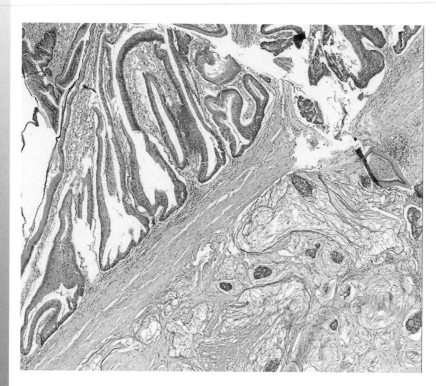

Fig. 25. Colloid carcinoma associated with an intestinal-type IPMN component (*top left*).

extracellular mucin but the large pools seen in colloid carcinoma are lacking. Because this entity is rare,[34] metastases from other more common signet cell carcinomas, mammary or gastric, should be ruled out.[35]

HEPATOID CARCINOMA

Hepatoid carcinomas are an extremely rare malignant epithelial neoplasm, characterized by significant hepatocellular differentiation.[36,37] They can occur in pure form or are associated with conventional PDAC.[38,39] Hepatocellular carcinomas are composed of large polygonal cells with abundant eosinophilic cytoplasm. Bile production has been described as well as the presence of intracytoplasmic hyaline globules.[40] Immunohistochemistry for Hep Par 1, polyclonal CEA, and CD10 can be useful for diagnosis.[7]

MEDULLARY CARCINOMA

Medullary carcinoma is a neoplasm characterized by poor differentiation, a syncytial growth pattern, well-defined expanding borders, and high mitotic rates (**Fig. 28**A, B). Occasionally, a rich number of tumor-infiltrating CD3-positive lymphocytes are present, but in contrast to other medullary carcinomas, they lack a prominent Crohn-like lymphoid infiltrate (see **Fig. 28**C). Most medullary carcinomas are microsatellite unstable and this can easily be appreciated by immunohistochemistry for MLH1 and MSH2.[41,42] Most are wild-type *KRAS* gene and some have *BRAF* gene mutations. Patients with medullary carcinomas are more likely to have a family history of cancer and genetic counseling may be indicated. Despite their poor differentiation, they seem to have a better prognosis and they may not respond to 5-fluorouracil.[43,44]

UNDIFFERENTIATED CARCINOMA

Undifferentiated carcinomas are an epithelial neoplasm without a definite direction of differentiation. They can occur ex novo or be associated with other pancreatic neoplasms. They are usually large and widely invasive and any portion of the pancreas can be affected. The spectrum of morphology varies from highly cellular, pleomorphic epithelioid mononuclear cells with abundant cytoplasm, often admixed with bizarre multinucleated giant cells, to relatively monomorphic epithelioid and spindle cells (**Fig. 29**A).[7,45] The necrosis is usually extensive. Cytokeratins are expressed

Fig. 26. Colloid carcinoma. The neoplastic epithelial component is immunoreactive for MUC2 (*A*) and CDX2 (*B*).

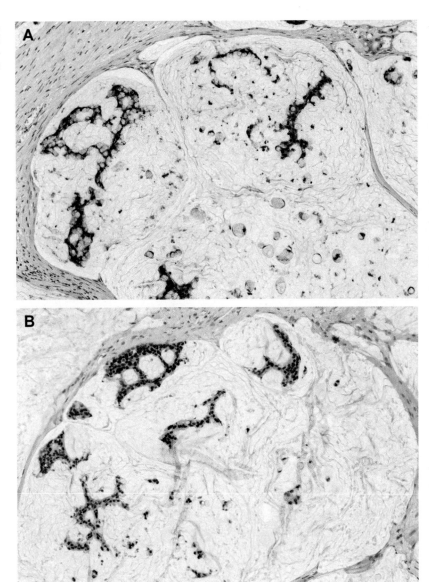

in more than 80% of cases (see **Fig. 29**B), although they may be focal; most express vimentin, focal actin, and MUC1.[46] At the molecular level, they are characterized by loss of E-cadherin and dysregulated β-catenin expression that seems related to the poor cohesiveness and loss of differentiation.[47] The genetic mutations parallel those of ductal adenocarcinoma and when both ductal and undifferentiated elements are present, they have the same *KRAS* mutations.[46] The prognosis is poor, with a mean survival of 5 months.

UNDIFFERENTIATED CARCINOMA WITH OSTEOCLAST-LIKE GIANT CELLS

Undifferentiated carcinomas with osteoclast-like giant cells are a rare neoplasm composed of highly atypical mononuclear pleomorphic cells and benign-appearing multinucleated giant cells (**Fig. 30**A). Many of these arise in association with a noninvasive precursor neoplasm, such as MCN. Molecular analysis has established that the multinucleated giant cells represent a reactive, non-neoplastic component.[48–50] The osteoclast-like

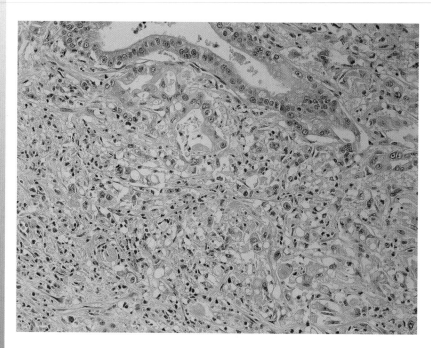

Fig. 27. Signet ring cell carcinoma with noncohesive cells associated with focal tubular component.

giant cells do not show mitotic activity. In some carcinomas, osteoid or osseous formation can be observed. The osteoclast-like giant cells express CD68 (see **Fig. 30B**), vimentin, and CD45 but not cytokeratins.[51] Mononuclear cells can be categorized as atypical or histiocyte-like.[7] The atypical mononuclear cells almost always express vimentin whereas only a minority express cytokeratin. Although it was initially thought that this neoplasm was less aggressive because of occasional cases of long survival rates, recent studies have shown a poor prognosis.[7,52]

DIFFERENTIAL DIAGNOSIS

Non-neoplastic mimickers of PDAC (discussed elsewhere in this issue) mostly fall into the category of inflammatory and fibrotic conditions correlated in various ways with CP.

CHRONIC PANCREATITIS

The macroscopic distinction of CP from PDAC may be difficult. In alcoholic CP, the scarring areas, with the exception of late stage, are intermixed with preserved lobular parenchyma; calculi as well as extrapancreatic pseudocyst can be observed.[53] Whenever present, the stenosis of the bile duct is not abrupt but shows a tapering appearance.[54]

The crucial components of CP are chronic inflammation, pancreatic fibrosis, acinar atrophy, and duct dilatation and obstruction.[8,55,56] There is a generalized involvement of the glands with interlobular fibrosis, which in long-standing cases is increasingly accompanied by intralobular fibrosis. With the progressive loss of the acinar cell component, the pancreatic lobule, which still retains its lobular architecture, is characterized by central ducts surrounded by clusters of ductules (**Fig. 31**). In advanced fibrotic stages, the

 Differential Diagnosis
CHRONIC PANCREATITIS

Features suggestive for PDAC

1. Haphazardly distributed neoplastic glands

2. Presence of perineural, vascular, or extrapancreatic tissue invasion

3. Glands next to muscular arteries or naked ducts in the adipose tissue

4. Nuclear variation greater than 4:1 from cell to cell within a gland

5. Prominent multiple nucleoli

6. Intraluminal necrosis

7. Incomplete glands

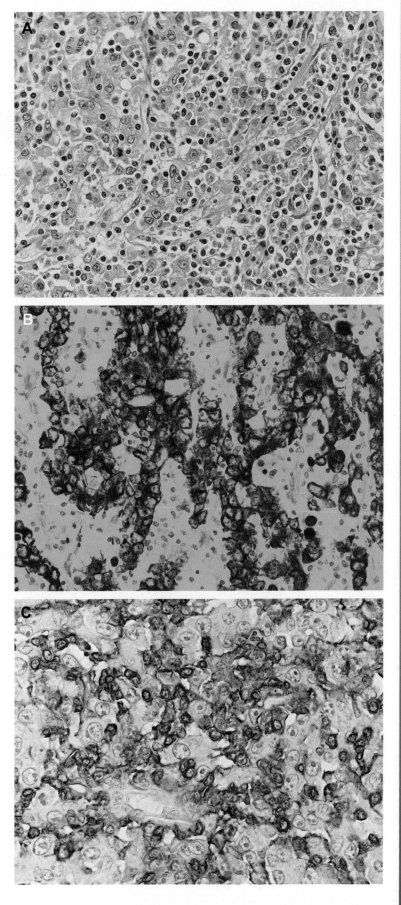

Fig. 28. Medullary carcinoma with syncytial growth pattern. (*A*) Hematoxylin-eosin, (*B*) keratin immunoreactivity, and (*C*) peritumoral and intratumoral CD3-positive T lymphocytes.

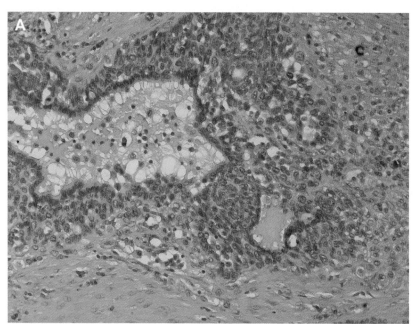

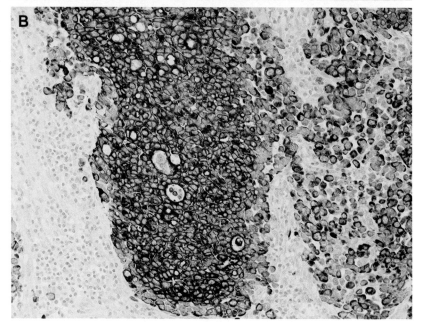

Fig. 29. Undifferentiated carcinoma characterized by epithelioid and spindle cells. (*A*) Hematoxylin-eosin and (*B*) keratin immuno-reactivity.

elements that remain are the islets. They usually aggregate together in pseudonodular formations, resulting in an apparent increase in mass or adenomatoid changes, and may occasionally show pseudoperineural invasion for their close relationship with nerves. Endocrine cell clusters can be observed within the adipose tissue. Alternatively, with the naked ducts, the latter phenomenon does not reflect true proliferation and adipose tissue infiltration but rather the result of a marked fibroadipose transformation of the pancreatic parenchyma simulating adipose tissue infiltration. Immunohistochemistry can be useful for demonstrating the preservation of

Fig. 30. Undifferentiated carcinoma with osteoclast-like giant cells with multinucleated giant cells associated with mononuclear cells. (*A*) Hematoxylin-eosin and (*B*) osteoclast-like giant cells immunoreactive for CD68.

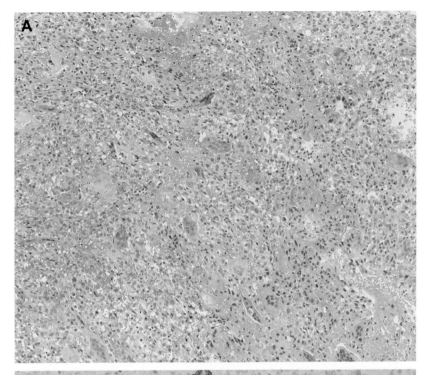

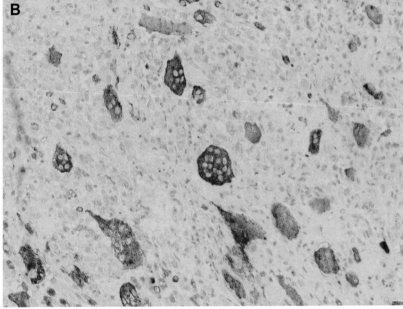

the lobular architecture of the pancreas and for demonstrating the endocrine nature of the round cell clusters in perineural spaces or in apparently inappropriate locations within the adipose tissue.

The most helpful microscopic findings in distinguishing a well-differentiated PDAC from reactive glands are the distribution, location, architecture, and cytologic features.[7,8,56]

AUTOIMMUNE PANCREATITIS

AIP deserves special attention in the differential diagnosis of PDAC.[57] AIP is now considered

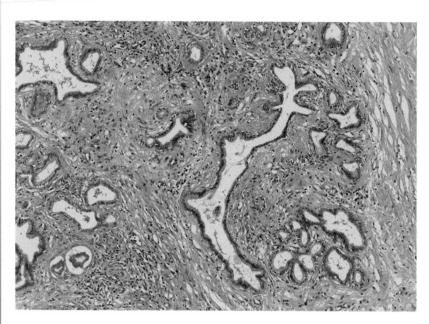

Fig. 31. Tubular complexes in CP, characterized by a central duct surrounded by small ducts.

the pancreatic manifestation of a systemic fibroinflammatory disease in which affected extrapancreatic organs also demonstrate a lymphoplasmacytic infiltration with abundant IgG4-positive plasma cells.[58,59] Clinically, radiographically, and grossly, the disease most commonly mimics pancreatic carcinoma because it predominantly affects the pancreatic head and the bile duct.[60–64] Histologically, however, it is not difficult to distinguish from ductal adenocarcinoma of the pancreas or other pancreatic malignancies. The microscopic features of AIP are dominated by lymphoplasmacytic periductal infiltration, storiform fibrosis, and venulitis.[65–67] In approximately 40% of patients, a peculiar granulocytic infiltration of the epithelial duct, termed, *granulocytic epithelial lesion (GEL)*, has been reported.[68]

Two main subtypes with differing clinicopathologic features can be distinguished:

1. Lymphoplasmacytic sclerosing pancreatitis (LPSP)-AIP without GELs (synonyms: lymphoplasmacytic sclerosing pancreatitis, lobulocentric pancreatitis, and GEL-negative pancreatitis): characterized by prominent lymphoplasmacytic infiltrate surrounding small-sized interlobular pancreatic ducts, storiform fibrosis, and obliterative phlebitis; GELs are typically absent.[55,61,67,69] Immunostaining reveals abundant (>10 cells/high-power field [HPF]) IgG4-positive cells.
2. Idiopathic duct-centric pancreatitis (IDCP)-AIP with GELs (synonyms: ductocentric pancreatitis

and GEL-positive pancreatitis): shares some features with LPSP although they are less prominent. The most distinctive feature is the presence of GELs.[68] The other distinctive feature is the scanty presence (<10 cells/hpf) or complete absence of IgG4-positive plasma cells on immunostaining.[69,70]

PARADUODENAL PANCREATITIS

Paraduodenal pancreatitis (synonyms: groove pancreatitis and cystic dystrophy of duodenal wall) may simulate PDAC, clinically and macroscopically. The majority of cases present with a stenosis of the second portion of the duodenum, with multiple cysts within a thickened duodenal wall and with variable extension to the groove compressing the common bile duct.[9,71–75] Histologically, paraduodenal pancreatitis is characterized by inflammatory, cystic, and fibrotic changes that develop within a intraduodenal pancreatic tissue associated to the minor papilla.[9,74]

NEOPLASTIC MIMICKERS OF PDAC

AMPULLARY CARCINOMA

Ampullary carcinoma, a tumor centered in the region of the ampulla of Vater, represents 5% of all gastrointestinal tumors but accounts for up to 36% of the surgically operable pancreatoduodenal tumors.[76] The unequivocal establishment of ampullary origin is possible in small lesions by applying strict topographic criteria during the gross and histologic examination and by the recognition of preinvasive modification in the anatomic structures of the ampulla.[77] The clinical importance of differentiating ampullary cancer from PDAC lies in its significantly better prognosis.

PANCREATIC INTRAEPITHELIAL NEOPLASIA

PanIN is a microscopic papillary or flat noninvasive epithelial neoplasm arising in the pancreatic ducts. PanINs are characterized by columnar to cuboidal cells with varying amounts of mucin and degrees of cytologic and architectural atypia. The high-grade PanIN-3 shares with the invasive glands of a conventional PDAC severe cytologic and architectural atypia (**Fig. 32**).[78] The distinction is based on the evaluation of the number, distribution, and locations of the glands. The presence of a desmoplastic stroma around the ducts is suggestive of invasive carcinoma (**Fig. 33**).[2,7]

INTRADUCTAL PAPILLARY MUCINOUS NEOPLASMS

IPMNs are grossly visible (typically >1 cm) intraductal proliferation of columnar mucin-producing cells, arising in the main pancreatic duct or its major branches. They form a heterogeneous group of neoplasms, which can be divided into different types on the basis of their morphology and mucin immunophenotype.[7,79–81]

MUCINOUS CYSTIC NEOPLASMS

MCNs are well-circumscribed cystic lesions that affect almost exclusively women, predominantly involve the tail of the pancreas, and do not communicate with the ductal system. They present with a characteristic subepithelial ovarian-type stroma.[7,82]

Their differential diagnosis with PDAC is mainly based on clinical, radiologic, and macroscopic features. A careful examination and an extensive sampling of the lesions are crucial for the detection of an invasive adenocarcinoma component. The prognosis for those invasive carcinomas associated with IPMNs and MCNs is better than that for conventional PDAC.[7]

SOLID CELLULAR PANCREATIC NEOPLASMS

Solid cellular pancreatic neoplasms are a group of pancreatic neoplasms that share a higher cellularity, great dimensions, and pushing margins. The most common types are endocrine neoplasms, solid pseudopapillary neoplasms, and acinar carcinomas (discussed elsewhere in this issue).

ENDOCRINE NEOPLASMS

A preoperative diagnosis of endocrine neoplasm can be made by FNA cytology. The smears are

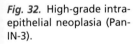

Fig. 32. High-grade intraepithelial neoplasia (PanIN-3).

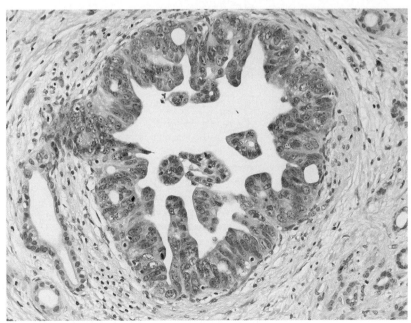

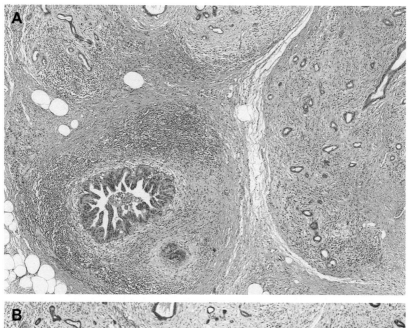

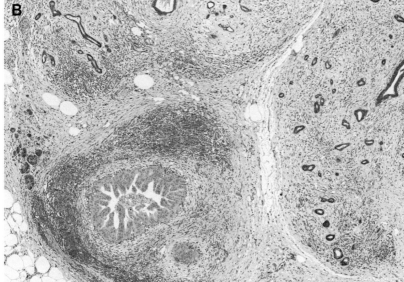

Fig. 33. Infiltrative ductal adenocarcinoma (*bottom left*) associated with atrophic lobuli. (*A*) Hematoxylin-eosin and (*B*) DPC4 immunostaining with loss of reactivity in the neoplastic duct and preserved immunolabeling in the ducts of atrophic lobuli.

hypercellular with a clean background, except for high-grade neoplasia. The cells can be individually dispersed or arranged in clusters. The nuclei are frequently uniform, round to oval, with a salt and pepper pattern (coarse, finely distributed chromatin) but sometimes they can be pleomorphic and hyperchromatic.

In histologic sections, the lack of desmoplastic stroma, the organoid pattern, the cytologic features, and the lack of mitotic activity are diagnostically helpful. The diagnosis can be confirmed by the immunoreactivity for chromogranin and synaptophysin.

SOLID PSEUDOPAPILLARY TUMOR

A preoperative diagnosis of solid pseudopapillary tumor can usually be made by FNA cytology. The cytologic smears are highly cellular and characterized by the presence of branching papillae, formed by delicate central fibrovascular stalks covered by one or more layers of mild atypical, monomorphous cells. The cytoplasm is eosinophilic, and the nuclei are round, oval nuclei with grooves and finely granular chromatin. Eosinophilic, hyaline globules, and numerous foam cells may also be present.

Histologically, solid pseudopapillary tumors have a distinct appearance and the differential diagnosis with PDAC is usually easy. Immunohistochemistry can help in the differential diagnosis, showing positivity for vimentin, CD56, CD10, and neuron-specific enolase, whereas the immunoreactivity for broad-spectrum keratin markers, CAM 5.2 and KL1, is usually negative. The abnormal nuclear positivity for β-catenin supports the diagnosis.[7]

ACINAR CELL CARCINOMA

In acinar cell carcinoma, aspirate smears show loosely cohesive groups of cells that show the typical acinar differentiation with a cytoplasm filled with deeply eosinophilic granules. The cells show signs of atypia, with prominent nucleoli and mitoses; necrotic debris is frequently found. An endocrine cell component may be present.

Histologically, the differential diagnosis with PDAC is easy. In difficult cases, the immunohistochemical positivity for trypsin and the negativity for carcinoma markers are diagnostically helpful. The neuroendocrine markers may be present in a minor component of cells.

METASTASES

Many extrapancreatic epithelial and nonepithelial neoplasms can metastasize to the pancreas. The most common metastatic malignancies to the pancreas are renal cell carcinomas, melanomas, colorectal carcinomas, breast carcinomas, and sarcomas.[83] Patient history, morphology, and immunohistochemical markers can be useful in establishing a diagnosis.

DIAGNOSIS

Although a correct diagnosis is mandatory for planning the therapeutic approach and establishing a prognosis, accurate preoperative diagnosis sometimes is difficult to achieve. The ideal diagnostic test, as in other disease, should be the tissue diagnosis with a Tru-Cut biopsy, because the tissue can also be used for ancillary studies. Unfortunately, diagnostic pancreatic tissue biopsies are not always available. The less-invasive methods, such as FNA cytology with ultrasound guidance or endoscopic ultrasound (EUS)-guided biopsies, have a better level of safety and are considered reliable in detecting the presence of

malignant cells. The sensitivity and specificity reported by expert teams are 69% and 100%, respectively.[84,85] The sensitivity and specificity of EUS with FNA are greater than 90% and 100%, respectively.[86] Direct bile duct or pancreatic duct brushing cytology can also be performed; the low sensitivity, approximately 50%, depends on the frequent reported sampling errors, due both to the lack of direct visualization of the lesions and the secondary associated reactive epithelia.[87,88] An increased sensitivity for the detection of malignancy have been reported with the ThinPrep (Cytyc) technique.[89]

Independently, on the used sampling method, the accuracy of diagnosis is higher when a close working relationship is present among clinicians, radiologists, and pathologists. On-site interpretation makes it possible either to discontinue the procedure once diagnostic material is obtained or to obtain additional material.[84,90–92]

Whether or not a lesion should be punctured depends on many different aspects, most of them clinical and radiologic. In many centers, if a mass is resectable, surgeons perform a pancreatectomy because of the false-negative results with both cytology and biopsy (10% to 30%).[93] For that reason, approximately 5% to 10% of pancreatectomies performed with the clinicoradiologic suspicion of cancer prove to be non-neoplastic masses (pseudotumors).[8,81] A morphologic diagnosis has to be served to all patients, either on the primary or secondary lesions, before planning chemotherapy.

The pitfalls that pathologists have to avoid in the interpretation of both cytology and biopsy are many. The best way to avoid them is to know them. The answer to the question, What should pathologists know? is that they should know all the clinical and radiologic relevant features. The most important differential diagnosis of ductal carcinoma is CP,[94] especially tumor-forming pancreatitis, such as AIP.[8,94,95] Recognition of gastric and duodenal epithelial contamination is the most important element to be considered in the EUS-guided FNA cytology, especially in the differential diagnosis of mucin-secreting low-grade neoplasms. Overdiagnosis of carcinoma has to be avoided in the presence of cellular atypia due to gastritis or duodenitis.

In ductal carcinoma, cytologic smears are characterized by high cellularity and the presence of relatively pure neoplastic cellular component. The presence of normal ductular-like aggregates serves by comparison. Major criteria of malignancy are considered—the presence of nuclear crowding and overlapping, the irregular chromatin distribution, and the irregular nuclear contour—whereas minor criteria are nuclear enlargement, presence of single malignant cells, necrosis, and mitosis.[92]

In biopsy interpretation of a primary pancreatic lesion, the following features are helpful in the differential diagnosis with CP[2,8,56]:

- Loss of original lobular structure of the pancreatic tissue, resulting in a haphazard distribution of glands
- Variation in nuclear area greater than 4:1 from cell to cell
- Prominent and multiple nucleoli
- Presence of incomplete glands, intraluminal necrosis
- Glands immediately adjacent to muscular artery
- Perineural invasion by glands and vascular invasion.

In differential diagnosis with AIP, the presence of elevated serum IgG4 level and dense IgG4-positive plasma cell infiltration in tissue specimens (more than 20 to 50 cells per HPF) have been reported in 50% to 60% of cases whereas the IgG4-negative cases show GELs.[9,68,70]

PROGNOSIS

The poor survival of patients with PDAC depends on the fact that almost all patients have metastatic disease at diagnosis. Autopsy studies demonstrated that 30% of patients die with locally destructive disease, without or with minimal metastatic disease, and 70% die with widespread metastatic disease.[96] The overall 5-year survival rate of patients is 3% to 5%.[4,97] Untreated patients have a mean survival time of 3 to 5 months and a 5-year survival rate close to 0%. Although, chemotherapy may improve long-term survival outcome,[98,99] the most important factor in determining prognosis is resectability.[100,101]

Stage is the main prognostic indicator in resected patients. Pancreatic cancers are staged according to the 7th edition of TNM system.[102] Survival is best in patients with small carcinomas (<3 cm) and negative lymph nodes, with a 5-year survival rate approaching 40%.[42]

The involvement of the retroperitoneal margin is one of the most important predictor factors.[103,104] Patients with pathologically negative resection margins (R0) have a median survival of 1.3 years[105] and a 5-year survival of 15% to 20%.[106] Campbell and colleagues[107] have reported that the presence of microscopic tumor involvement within 1 mm of retroperitoneal resection margin should be considered synonymous with incomplete excision and classified as R1 (**Fig. 34**). Lymph node status is related to survival and seems to predict long-term survival.[108] The lymph node ratio, that is, the ratio of the number of metastatic nodes to the total number of nodes examined, is one of the most powerful predictors of survival after surgery.[109,110] Other reported poor prognostic indicators include tumor grade,[16] mitotic index,

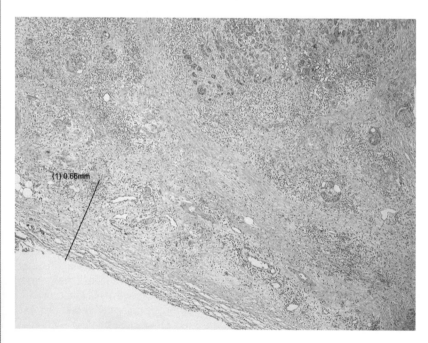

Fig. 34. Infiltrating ductal adenocarcinoma with neoplastic cells close (0.66 mm) to the retroperitoneal resection margin.

major vessel involvement, and vascular and perineural invasion.[111,112]

At the molecular level, the divergent patterns of failure and locally destructive versus widespread metastatic disease have been correlated with distinct genetic alterations. Smad4/DPC4 gene inactivation is associated with poorer prognosis in patients with surgically resected cancers. Patients with wild-type Smad4/DPC4 have a medial survival time of 14.2 months whereas patients with genetically inactivated Smad4/DPC4 gene have a medial survival time of 11.5 months.[113] The loss of DPC4 expression at the immunohistochemical level has been found in 75% and 22% of patients with widespread and prevalently locally destructive pancreatic cancers, respectively.[114]

REFERENCES

1. Bolender RP. Stereological study of pancreatic exocrine cells. Adv Cytopharmacol 1974;2: 99–106.
2. Hruban RH, Fukushima N. Pancreatic adenocarcinoma: update on the surgical pathology of carcinomas of ductal origin and PanINs. Mod Pathol 2007;20(Suppl 1):S61–70.
3. Pour PM. The silent killer. Int J Pancreatol 1991; 10(2):103–4.
4. Jemal A, Thun MJ, Ries LA, et al. Annual report to the nation on the status of cancer, 1975–2005, featuring trends in lung cancer, tobacco use, and tobacco control. J Natl Cancer Inst 2008;100(23): 1672–94.
5. AIRT. (Italian Association Tumor Registries). Italian Cancer Figures-Report-2006. Epidemiol Prev 2006;30(1):46–7.
6. Quirke P. The pathologist, the surgeon and colorectal cancer—get it right because it matters. In: Kirkhan NR, editor. Progress in pathology. Edinburgh, London; New York: Churchill Livingstone; 1998. p. 201–13.
7. Hruban RH, Pitman MB, Klimstra DS. Tumors of the pancreas. AFIP Atlas of tumor pathology, vol. 6. Washington, DC: American Registry of Pathology, Armed Forces Institute of Pathology; 2007.
8. Adsay NV, Bandyopadhyay S, Basturk O, et al. Chronic pancreatitis or pancreatic ductal adenocarcinoma? Semin Diagn Pathol 2004;21(4):268–76.
9. Zamboni G, Capelli P, Scarpa A, et al. Nonneoplastic mimickers of pancreatic neoplasms. Arch Pathol Lab Med 2009;133(3):439–53.
10. Luttges J, Zamboni G, Kloppel G. Recommendation for the examination of pancreaticoduodenectomy specimens removed from patients with carcinoma of the exocrine pancreas. A proposal for a standardized pathological staging of pancreaticoduodenectomy specimens including a checklist. Dig Surg 1999;16(4):291–6.
11. Zamboni G, Capelli P, Pesci A, et al. Pancreatic head mass: what can be done? Classification: the pathological point of view. JOP 2000;1(3 Suppl): 77–84.
12. Westra WH, Hruban RH, Phelps TH, et al. Surgical pathology dissection: an illustrated guide. 2nd edition. New York: Springer; 2003.
13. Costa J. Benign epithelial inclusions in pancreatic nerves. Am J Clin Pathol 1977;67(3):306–7.
14. Klöppel G, Hruban R, Longnecker D, et al. Ductal adenocarcinoma of the pancreas. In: Hamilton SR, Aaltonen LA, editors. Tumours of the digestive system. World Health Organization classification of tumors. Pathology and genetics. Lyon (France): IARC Press; 2000.
15. Klöppel G, Lingenthal G, von Bülow M, et al. Histological and fine structural features of pancreatic ductal adenocarcinomas in relation to growth and prognosis. Histopathology 1985;9:841–56.
16. Luttges J, Schemm S, Vogel I, et al. The grade of pancreatic ductal carcinoma is an independent prognostic factor and is superior to the immunohistochemical assessment of proliferation. J Pathol 2000;191(2):154–61.
17. Adsay NV, Basturk O, Bonnett M, et al. A proposal for a new and more practical grading scheme for pancreatic ductal adenocarcinoma. Am J Surg Pathol 2005;29(6):724–33.
18. Adsay V, Logani S, Sarkar F, et al. Foamy gland pattern of pancreatic ductal adenocarcinoma: a deceptively benign-appearing variant. Am J Surg Pathol 2000;24(4):493–504.
19. Luttges J, Vogel I, Menke M, et al. Clear cell carcinoma of the pancreas: an adenocarcinoma with ductal phenotype. Histopathology 1998;32(5): 444–8.
20. Kosmahl M, Pauser U, Anlauf M, et al. Pancreatic ductal adenocarcinomas with cystic features: neither rare nor uniform. Mod Pathol 2005;18(9): 1157–64.
21. Kardon DE, Thompson LD, Przygodzki RM, et al. Adenosquamous carcinoma of the pancreas: a clinicopathologic series of 25 cases. Mod Pathol 2001; 14(5):443–51.
22. Hsu JT, Yeh CN, Chen YR, et al. Adenosquamous carcinoma of the pancreas. Digestion 2005; 72(2–3):104–8.
23. Ishikawa O, Matzui Y, Aoki I, et al. Adenosquamous carcinoma of the pancreas: a clinicopathologic study and report of three cases. Cancer 1980;46: 1192–6.
24. Madura JA, Jarman BT, Doherty MG, et al. Adenosquamous carcinoma of the pancreas. Arch Surg 1999;134(6):599–603.

25. Brennan MF, Moccia RD, Klimstra D. Management of adenocarcinoma of the body and tail of the pancreas. Ann Surg 1996;223(5):506–11 [discussion: 511–2].

26. Brody JR, Costantino CL, Potoczek M, et al. Adenosquamous carcinoma of the pancreas harbors KRAS2, DPC4 and TP53 molecular alterations similar to pancreatic ductal adenocarcinoma. Mod Pathol 2009;22(5):651–9.

27. Voong KR, Davison J, Pawlik TM, et al. Resected pancreatic adenosquamous carcinoma: clinicopathologic review and evaluation of adjuvant chemotherapy and radiation in 38 patients. Hum Pathol 2010;41(1):113–22.

28. Itani KM, Karni A, Green L. Squamous cell carcinoma of the pancreas. J Gastrointest Surg 1999; 3(5):512–5.

29. Adsay NV, Pierson C, Sarkar F, et al. Colloid (mucinous noncystic) carcinoma of the pancreas. Am J Surg Pathol 2001;25(1):26–42.

30. Adsay NV, Conlon KC, Zee SY, et al. Intraductal papillary-mucinous neoplasms of the pancreas: an analysis of in situ and invasive carcinomas in 28 patients. Cancer 2002;94(1):62–77.

31. Seidel G, Zahurak M, Iacobuzio-Donahue C, et al. Almost all infiltrating colloid carcinomas of the pancreas and periampullary region arise from in situ papillary neoplasms: a study of 39 cases. Am J Surg Pathol 2002;26(1):56–63.

32. Adsay NV, Merati K, Nassar H, et al. Pathogenesis of colloid (pure mucinous) carcinoma of exocrine organs: coupling of gel-forming mucin (MUC2) production with altered cell polarity and abnormal cell-stroma interaction may be the key factor in the morphogenesis and indolent behavior of colloid carcinoma in the breast and pancreas. Am J Surg Pathol 2003;27(5):571–8.

33. Tracey KJ, O'Brien MJ, Williams LF, et al. Signet ring carcinoma of the pancreas, a rare variant with very high CEA values. Immunohistologic comparison with adenocarcinoma. Dig Dis Sci 1984;29(6):573–6.

34. Chow LT, Chow WH. Signet-ring mucinous adenocarcinoma of the pancreas. Chin Med Sci J 1994; 9(3):176–8.

35. Stokes MB, Kumar A, Symmans WF, et al. Pancreatic endocrine tumor with signet ring cell features: a case report with novel ultrastructural observations. Ultrastruct Pathol 1998;22(2):147–52.

36. Yano T, Ishikura H, Wada T, et al. Hepatoid adenocarcinoma of the pancreas. Histopathology 1999; 35(1):90–2.

37. Paner GP, Thompson KS, Reyes CV. Hepatoid carcinoma of the pancreas. Cancer 2000;88(7): 1582–9.

38. Cuilliere P, Lazure T, Bui M, et al. Solid adenoma with exclusive hepatocellular differentiation: a new variant among pancreatic benign neoplasms? Virchows Arch 2002;441(5):519–22.

39. Hruban RH, Molina JM, Reddy MN, et al. A neoplasm with pancreatic and hepatocellular differentiation presenting with subcutaneous fat necrosis. Am J Clin Pathol 1987;88(5):639–45.

40. Hameed O, Xu H, Saddeghi S, et al. Hepatoid carcinoma of the pancreas: a case report and literature review of a heterogeneous group of tumors. Am J Surg Pathol 2007;31(1):146–52.

41. Wilentz RE, Goggins M, Redston M, et al. Genetic, immunohistochemical, and clinical features of medullary carcinoma of the pancreas: a newly described and characterized entity. Am J Pathol 2000;156(5):1641–51.

42. Goggins M, Offerhaus GJ, Hilgers W, et al. Pancreatic adenocarcinomas with DNA replication errors (RER+) are associated with wild-type K-ras and characteristic histopathology. Poor differentiation, a syncytial growth pattern, and pushing borders suggest RER+. Am J Pathol 1998; 152(6):1501–7.

43. Hruban RH, Adsay NV. Molecular classification of neoplasms of the pancreas. Hum Pathol 2009; 40(5):612–23.

44. Ribic CM, Sargent DJ, Moore MJ, et al. Tumor microsatellite-instability status as a predictor of benefit from fluorouracil-based adjuvant chemotherapy for colon cancer. N Engl J Med 2003; 349(3):247–57.

45. Kuroda N, Sawada T, Miyazaki E, et al. Anaplastic carcinoma of the pancreas with rhabdoid features. Pathol Int 2000;50(1):57–62.

46. Paal E, Thompson LD, Frommelt RA, et al. A clinicopathologic and immunohistochemical study of 35 anaplastic carcinomas of the pancreas with a review of the literature. Ann Diagn Pathol 2001;5(3):129–40.

47. Winter JM, Ting AH, Vilardell F, et al. Absence of E-cadherin expression distinguishes noncohesive from cohesive pancreatic cancer. Clin Cancer Res 2008;14(2):412–8.

48. Gocke CD, Dabbs DJ, Benko FA, et al. KRAS oncogene mutations suggest a common histogenetic origin for pleomorphic giant cell tumor of the pancreas, osteoclastoma of the pancreas, and pancreatic duct adenocarcinoma. Hum Pathol 1997;28(1):80–3.

49. Westra WH, Sturm P, Drillenburg P, et al. K-ras oncogene mutations in osteoclast-like giant cell tumors of the pancreas and liver: genetic evidence to support origin from the duct epithelium. Am J Surg Pathol 1998;22(10):1247–54.

50. Sakai Y, Kupelioglu AA, Yanagisawa A, et al. Origin of giant cells in osteoclast-like giant cell tumors of the pancreas. Hum Pathol 2000;31(10): 1223–9.

51. Deckard-Janatpour K, Kragel S, Teplitz RL, et al. Tumors of the pancreas with osteoclast-like and pleomorphic giant cells: an immunohistochemical and ploidy study. Arch Pathol Lab Med 1998; 122(3):266–72.

52. Solcia E, Capella C, Klöppel G. 3rd edition. Tumors of the pancreas. AFIP Atlas of tumor pathology, vol. 20. Washington, DC: Armed Forces Institute of Pathology; 1997.

53. Kloppel G, Maillet AB. Pseudocyst in chronic pancreatitis: a morphological analysis of 57 resection specimens and 9 autopsy pancreata. Pancreas 1991;6:266–74.

54. Kloppel G. Chronic pancreatitis of alcoholic and nonalcoholic origin. Semin Diagn Pathol 2004; 21(4):227–36.

55. Kloppel G. Chronic pancreatitis, pseudotumors and other tumor-like lesions. Mod Pathol 2007; 20(Suppl 1):S113–31.

56. Kloppel G, Adsay NV. Chronic pancreatitis and the differential diagnosis versus pancreatic cancer. Arch Pathol Lab Med 2009;133(3):382–7.

57. Ito T, Nakano I, Koyanagi S, et al. Autoimmune pancreatitis as a new clinical entity. Three cases of autoimmune pancreatitis with effective steroid therapy. Dig Dis Sci 1997;42(7):1458–68.

58. Kamisawa T, Funata N, Hayashi Y. Lymphoplasmacytic sclerosing pancreatitis is a pancreatic lesion of IgG4-related systemic disease. Am J Surg Pathol 2004;28(8):1114.

59. Okazaki K. Is IgG4-associated multifocal systemic fibrosis the same disease entity as autoimmune pancreatitis? Intern Med 2007;46(3):117–8.

60. Pearson RK, Longnecker DS, Chari ST, et al. Controversies in clinical pancreatology: autoimmune pancreatitis: does it exist? Pancreas 2003; 27(1):1–13.

61. Deshpande V, Mino-Kenudson M, Brugge W, et al. Autoimmune pancreatitis: more than just a pancreatic disease? A contemporary review of its pathology. Arch Pathol Lab Med 2005;129(9):1148–54.

62. Cavallini G, Frulloni L. Autoimmunity and chronic pancreatitis: a concealed relationship. JOP 2001; 2(2):61–8.

63. Frulloni L, Lunardi C, Simone R, et al. Identification of a novel antibody associated with autoimmune pancreatitis. N Engl J Med 2009;361(22):2135–42.

64. Frulloni L, Scattolini C, Falconi M, et al. Autoimmune pancreatitis: differences between the focal and diffuse forms in 87 patients. Am J Gastroenterol 2009;104(9):2288–94.

65. Kloppel G, Luttges J, Lohr M, et al. Autoimmune pancreatitis: pathological, clinical, and immunological features. Pancreas 2003;27(1):14–9.

66. Ectors N, Maillet B, Aerts R, et al. Non-alcoholic duct destructive chronic pancreatitis. Gut 1997; 41(2):263–8.

67. Notohara K, Burgart LJ, Yadav D, et al. Idiopathic chronic pancreatitis with periductal lymphoplasmacytic infiltration: clinicopathologic features of 35 cases. Am J Surg Pathol 2003;27(8): 1119–27.

68. Zamboni G, Luttges J, Capelli P, et al. Histopathological features of diagnostic and clinical relevance in autoimmune pancreatitis: a study on 53 resection specimens and 9 biopsy specimens. Virchows Arch 2004;445(6):552–63.

69. Sugumar A, Kloppel G, Chari ST. Autoimmune pancreatitis: pathologic subtypes and their implications for its diagnosis. Am J Gastroenterol 2009; 104(9):2308–10 [quiz: 2311].

70. Kojima M, Sipos B, Klapper W, et al. Autoimmune pancreatitis: frequency, IgG4 expression, and clonality of T and B cells. Am J Surg Pathol 2007;31(4): 521–8.

71. Potet F, Duclert N. Cystic dystrophy on aberrant pancreas of the duodenal wall. Arch Fr Mal App Dig 1970;59(4):223–38 [in French].

72. Stolte M, Weiss W, Volkholz H, et al. A special form of segmental pancreatitis. "Groove pancreatitis". Hepatogastroenterology 1982;29:198–208.

73. Yamaguchi K, Tanaka M. Groove pancreatitis masquerading as pancreatic carcinoma. Am J Surg 1992;163:312–8.

74. Adsay NV, Zamboni G. Paraduodenal pancreatitis: a clinico-pathologically distinct entity unifying "cystic dystrophy of heterotopic pancreas", "paraduodenal wall cyst", and "groove pancreatitis". Semin Diagn Pathol 2004;21(4):247–54.

75. Casetti L, Bassi C, Salvia R, et al. "Paraduodenal" pancreatitis: results of surgery on 58 consecutives patients from a single institution. World J Surg 2009;33(12):2664–9.

76. Yamaguchi K, Enjoji M. Carcinoma of the ampulla of vater. A clinicopathologic study and pathologic staging of 109 cases of carcinoma and 5 cases of adenoma. Cancer 1987;59(3):506–15.

77. Scarpa A, Capelli P, Zamboni G, et al. Neoplasia of the ampulla of Vater: Ki-ras and p53 mutations. Am J Pathol 1993;142:1163–72.

78. Hruban RH, Takaori K, Klimstra DS, et al. An illustrated consensus on the classification of pancreatic intraepithelial neoplasia and intraductal papillary mucinous neoplasms. Am J Surg Pathol 2004; 28(8):977–87.

79. Luttges J, Zamboni G, Longnecker D, et al. The immunohistochemical mucin expression pattern distinguishes different types of intraductal papillary mucinous neoplasms of the pancreas and determines their relationship to mucinous noncystic carcinoma and ductal adenocarcinoma. Am J Surg Pathol 2001;25(7):942–8.

80. Adsay NV, Merati K, Basturk O, et al. Pathologically and biologically distinct types of epithelium

in intraductal papillary mucinous neoplasms: delineation of an "intestinal" pathway of carcinogenesis in the pancreas. Am J Surg Pathol 2004;28(7): 839–48.

81. Abraham SC, Lee JH, Hruban RH, et al. Molecular and immunohistochemical analysis of intraductal papillary neoplasms of the biliary tract. Hum Pathol 2003;34(9):902–10.

82. Zamboni G, Scarpa A, Bogina G, et al. Mucinous cystic tumors of the pancreas: clinicopathological features, prognosis, and relationship to other mucinous cystic tumors. Am J Surg Pathol 1999; 23(4):410–22.

83. Reddy S, Edil BH, Cameron JL, et al. Pancreatic resection of isolated metastases from nonpancreatic primary cancers. Ann Surg Oncol 2008;15(11): 3199–206.

84. Ghaneh P, Costello E, Neoptolemos JP. Biology and management of pancreatic cancer. Gut 2007;56(8): 1134–52.

85. Bardales RH, Stelow EB, Mallery S, et al. Review of endoscopic ultrasound-guided fine-needle aspiration cytology. Diagn Cytopathol 2006; 34(2):140–75.

86. Raut CP, Grau AM, Staerkel GA, et al. Diagnostic accuracy of endoscopic ultrasound-guided fine-needle aspiration in patients with presumed pancreatic cancer. J Gastrointest Surg 2003;7(1): 118–26 [discussion: 127–8].

87. Logrono R, Kurtycz DF, Molina CP, et al. Analysis of false-negative diagnoses on endoscopic brush cytology of biliary and pancreatic duct strictures: the experience at 2 university hospitals. Arch Pathol Lab Med 2000;124(3):387–92.

88. Logrono R, Wong JY. Reporting the presence of significant epithelial atypia in pancreaticobiliary brush cytology specimens lacking evidence of obvious carcinoma: impact on performance measures. Acta Cytol 2004;48(5):613–21.

89. Volmar KE, Vollmer RT, Routbort MJ, et al. Pancreatic and bile duct brushing cytology in 1000 cases: review of findings and comparison of preparation methods. Cancer 2006;108(4):231–8.

90. Eloubeidi MA, Tamhane A, Jhala N, et al. Agreement between rapid onsite and final cytologic interpretations of EUS-guided FNA specimens: implications for the endosonographer and patient management. Am J Gastroenterol 2006;101(12): 2841–7.

91. Savides TJ, Donohue M, Hunt G, et al. EUS-guided FNA diagnostic yield of malignancy in solid pancreatic masses: a benchmark for quality performance measurement. Gastrointest Endosc 2007;66(2): 277–82.

92. Bellizzi AM, Stelow EB. Pancreatic cytopathology: a practical approach and review. Arch Pathol Lab Med 2009;133(3):388–404.

93. Isaacson R, Weiland LH, McIlrath DC. Biopsy of the pancreas. Arch Surg 1974;109(2):227–30.

94. Stelow EB, Bardales RH, Stanley MW. Pitfalls in endoscopic ultrasound-guided fine-needle aspiration and how to avoid them. Adv Anat Pathol Mar 2005;12(2):62–73.

95. Deshpande V, Mino-Kenudson M, Brugge WR, et al. Endoscopic ultrasound guided fine needle aspiration biopsy of autoimmune pancreatitis: diagnostic criteria and pitfalls. Am J Surg Pathol 2005; 29(11):1464–71.

96. Kamisawa T, Isawa T, Koike M, et al. Hematogenous metastases of pancreatic ductal carcinoma. Pancreas 1995;11(4):345–9.

97. Conlon KC, Klimstra DS, Brennan MF. Long-term survival after curative resection for pancreatic ductal adenocarcinoma. Clinicopathologic analysis of 5-year survivors. Ann Surg 1996;223(3): 273–9.

98. Oettle H, Post S, Neuhaus P, et al. Adjuvant chemotherapy with gemcitabine vs observation in patients undergoing curative-intent resection of pancreatic cancer: a randomized controlled trial. JAMA 2007;297(3):267–77.

99. Neoptolemos JP, Stocken DD, Friess H, et al. A randomized trial of chemoradiotherapy and chemotherapy after resection of pancreatic cancer. N Engl J Med 2004;350(12):1200–10.

100. Kuhlmann KF, de Castro SM, Wesseling JG, et al. Surgical treatment of pancreatic adenocarcinoma; actual survival and prognostic factors in 343 patients. Eur J Cancer 2004;40(4):549–58.

101. Neoptolemos JP, Stocken DD, Dunn JA, et al. Influence of resection margins on survival for patients with pancreatic cancer treated by adjuvant chemoradiation and/or chemotherapy in the ESPAC-1 randomized controlled trial. Ann Surg 2001;234(6):758–68.

102. Edge SB, Byrd DR, Compton CC, et al. AJCC cancer staging manual. 7th edition. New York: Springer; 2010.

103. Verbeke CS. Resection margins and R1 rates in pancreatic cancer–are we there yet? Histopathology 2008;52(7):787–96.

104. Verbeke CS, Menon KV. Variability in reporting resection margin status in pancreatic cancer. Ann Surg 2008;247(4):716–7.

105. Westgaard A, Tafjord S, Farstad IN, et al. Resectable adenocarcinomas in the pancreatic head: the retroperitoneal resection margin is an independent prognostic factor. BMC Cancer 2008;8:5.

106. Philip PA, Mooney M, Jaffe D, et al. Consensus report of the national cancer institute clinical trials planning meeting on pancreas cancer treatment. J Clin Oncol 2009;27(33):5660–9.

107. Campbell F, Smith RA, Whelan P, et al. Classification of R1 resections for pancreatic cancer: the prognostic relevance of tumour involvement within

1 mm of a resection margin. Histopathology 2009; 55(3):277–83.

108. Schnelldorfer T, Ware AL, Sarr MG, et al. Long-term survival after pancreatoduodenectomy for pancreatic adenocarcinoma: is cure possible? Ann Surg 2008;247(3):456–62.

109. Slidell MB, Chang DC, Cameron JL, et al. Impact of total lymph node count and lymph node ratio on staging and survival after pancreatectomy for pancreatic adenocarcinoma: a large, population-based analysis. Ann Surg Oncol 2008;15(1):165–74.

110. Pawlik TM, Gleisner AL, Cameron JL, et al. Prognostic relevance of lymph node ratio following pancreaticoduodenectomy for pancreatic cancer. Surgery 2007;141(5):610–8.

111. Ozaki H, Hiraoka T, Mizumoto R, et al. The prognostic significance of lymph node metastasis and intrapancreatic perineural invasion in pancreatic cancer after curative resection. Surg Today 1999; 29(1):16–22.

112. Mitsunaga S, Hasebe T, Kinoshita T, et al. Detail histologic analysis of nerve plexus invasion in invasive ductal carcinoma of the pancreas and its prognostic impact. Am J Surg Pathol 2007;31(11): 1636–44.

113. Blackford A, Serrano OK, Wolfgang CL, et al. SMAD4 gene mutations are associated with poor prognosis in pancreatic cancer. Clin Cancer Res 2009;15(14):4674–9.

114. Iacobuzio-Donahue CA, Fu B, Yachida S, et al. DPC4 gene status of the primary carcinoma correlates with patterns of failure in patients with pancreatic cancer. J Clin Oncol 2009;27(11): 1806–13.

PANCREATIC INTRAEPITHELIAL NEOPLASIA

Toby C. Cornish, MD, PhD, Ralph H. Hruban, MD*

KEYWORDS

- Pancreas • Pancreatic cancer precursors • Pancreatic intraepithelial neoplasia • PanIN
- Pancreatic ductal adenocarcinoma • Carcinogenesis • Lobulocentric atrophy
- Acinar ductal metaplasia

ABSTRACT

Pancreatic intraepithelial neoplasias (PanINs) are microscopic lesions of the pancreas. Traditionally viewed as a benign metaplasia of small ducts, evidence suggests that PanINs are neoplastic and that some PanINs progress to invasive ductal adenocarcinoma. The primary diagnostic challenge is distinguishing PanINs from other lesions, including invasive ductal adenocarcinoma, intraductal papillary mucinous neoplasm, and cancerization of benign ducts. PanINs are the most common of the pancreatic cancer precursor lesions, yet they remain poorly understood and are so small that they are almost clinically undetectable. Further study is required to define the role of PanINs in the carcinogenesis and early detection of pancreatic cancer.

Pathologic Key Features
PanIN

- PanINs are microscopic neoplastic lesions in smaller pancreatic ducts and are often associated with lobulocentric atrophy of the pancreas.

- PanIN-1 is flat (1A) or papillary (1B) with columnar epithelium and basally oriented, round nuclei.

- PanIN-2 is papillary with nuclear hyperchromasia, crowding, and pseudostratification.

- PanIN-3 is papillary, micropapillary, or cribriform with nuclear pleomorphism, frequent loss of nuclear orientation, and mitoses.

OVERVIEW: PANCREATIC DUCTAL ADENOCARCINOMA

Pancreatic ductal adenocarcinoma is among the deadliest of solid malignancies with a 5-year survival rate of less than 5%.[1] Although pancreatic cancer outcomes have improved little over the past 5 decades, mortality rates for other solid malignancies have decreased significantly. In breast and colon cancer, for example, this reduction is partially attributable to routine screening of high-risk populations for early curable preinvasive lesions. Like other carcinomas, pancreatic adenocarcinoma arises from distinct precursor lesions, including mucinous cystic neoplasms (MCNs), intraductal papillary mucinous neoplasms (IPMNs), and pancreatic intraepithelial neoplasias (PanINs). Unlike MCNs and IPMNs, both of which are macroscopic lesions, PanINs usually cannot be detected clinically, yet they are the most common precursors of invasive ductal adenocarcinoma. This has made PanINs a subject of significant interest in the early detection of pancreatic cancer.

Although PanINs have been recognized and described for over a century, consistent diagnostic

Disclosures: The authors have no relevant disclosures.
Department of Pathology, The Sol Goldman Pancreatic Cancer Research Center, The Johns Hopkins Medical Institutions, The Johns Hopkins Hospital, Weinberg Building, Room 2242, 401 North Broadway, Baltimore, MD 21231, USA
* Corresponding author.
E-mail address: rhruban@jhmi.edu

Surgical Pathology 4 (2011) 523–535
doi:10.1016/j.path.2011.03.005
1875-9181/11/$ – see front matter © 2011 Published by Elsevier Inc.

and grading criteria have only recently been introduced.[2–4] These diagnostic criteria adopted the PanIN nomenclature, uniting lesions previously described as ductal hyperplasia, metaplasia, proliferation, dysplasia, neoplasia, and carcinoma in situ. The prior lack of strict diagnostic criteria makes the early literature on these lesions difficult to interpret, but many studies clearly describe lesions now recognized as PanINs.

PanINs are common lesions and found in at least 16% of non-neoplastic pancreata.[5] Their abundance led many to conclude they are merely reactive metaplasia; however, clonal mutations in cancer-associated genes present in the majority of PanINs indicate they are true neoplastic lesions.[6] Like invasive ductal adenocarcinoma, PanINs increase in prevalence with increasing age.[5] The prevalence of PanINs also increases significantly in the settings of chronic pancreatitis (60% of pancreata with pancreatitis harbor a PanIN lesion) and invasive ductal adenocarcinoma (82%).[5] Most reports also indicate that, like invasive carcinoma, PanINs are more frequently found in the head of the pancreas.[5,7,8] Notably, although low-grade PanINs are commonly found in benign pancreata, high-grade lesions are significantly enriched in resections with pancreatic cancer, and PanIN-3, the highest grade of PanIN, is found almost exclusively in association with invasive ductal adenocarcinoma.[5] This suggests that low-grade PanINs (PanIN-1) either have a low rate of progression to high-grade lesions or that the PanIN-1 diagnostic category may be composed of a mixture of neoplastic and non-neoplastic lesions with an indistinguishable morphology. Terhune and colleagues, in a back-of-the-envelope calculation, estimated that the probability of a single PanIN progressing to invasive cancer is 0.86%.[9]

Several heritable conditions with a high risk of pancreatic cancer are also associated with an increase in PanINs. Familial pancreatic cancer patients (ie, individuals with at least 2 first-degree relatives with pancreatic cancer) who develop pancreatic cancer show an increased number of PanINs when compared with patients with sporadic pancreatic cancer. In familial pancreatic cancer patients, the overall PanIN frequency was 2.75-fold higher and the rate for PanIN-3 was 4.20-fold higher than in patients with pancreatic cancer but without a family history of the disease.[10] PanINs are also common in familial pancreatitis patients with confirmed PRSS1 mutations, because 77% of these patients have PanINs, and 50% of those with PanINs had a PanIN-3 lesion.[11]

GROSS FEATURES

PanINs are microscopic lesions, and pancreatic tissue bearing PanINs is usually grossly indistinguishable from pancreatic tissue containing only normal ducts. A notable but rare exception (discussed later) is PanIN associated with lobulocentric atrophy because the area of atrophy can occasionally be seen grossly as a fibrotic focus. These lesions are more likely to be grossly detectable if they are multifocal (**Fig. 1**).[12]

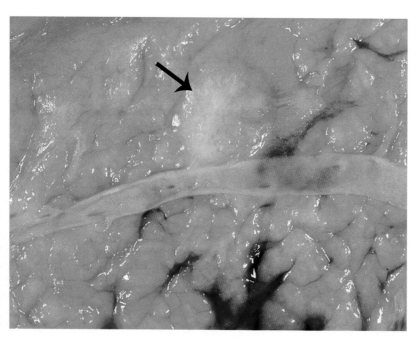

Fig. 1. The gross appearance of lobulocentric atrophy. PanINs are microscopic lesions involving small ducts and ductules and are not grossly visible; however, the lobulocentric atrophy that is often associated with PanINs can occasionally be visualized as a small, well-defined focus of fibrosis (*arrow*). The lesions can sometimes be detected on endoscopic ultrasound making lobulocentric atrophy a lesion of potential clinical importance.

MICROSCOPIC FEATURES

GENERAL FEATURES AND GRADING

PanINs are neoplastic lesions that replace the normal cuboidal epithelium of the pancreatic ducts and ductules. By definition, PanINs involve the smaller pancreatic ducts and ductules, and the majority are less than 5 mm in diameter. PanINs represent a continuum of dysplastic change and are graded morphologically based on the degree of cytologic and architectural atypia (**Fig. 2**).[3] There are 3 grades of PanIN with dysplastic features that range from negligible to the equivalent of carcinoma in situ.

PanIN-1 lesions (**Figs. 3** and **4**) are further classified as either flat (1A) or papillary (1B), but both have a tall columnar epithelium with basally oriented, round nuclei and abundant mucin. Because it is unclear that all pancreatic lesions with this morphology are true neoplasms, some pathologists prefer to use the term, PanIN/lesion or PanIN-1A/L, to describe these lesions. PanIN-2 lesions (**Fig. 5**) have papillary architecture and some nuclear dysplasia, including hyperchromasia, increased nuclear size, crowding, pseudostratification, and some loss of polarity. PanIN-3 lesions (**Fig. 6**) were previously called ductal carcinoma in situ. PanIN-3 has many of the features of invasive carcinoma, including a papillary, micropapillary, or cribriform architecture; pleomorphic nuclei; widespread loss of nuclear polarity; and occasional mitoses. PanIN-3 lesions are, however, noninvasive and remain confined by the basement membrane. Mucin is greatly reduced or absent, and dystrophic goblet cells may be present.

UNCOMMON VARIANTS OF PanIN

Three rare variants of PanIN are described in the literature: (1) intestinal variant, (2) oncocytic variant, and (3) foamy gland variant. These variants have a unique morphology and a characteristic mucin phenotype (discussed later); however, they have no known biologic or clinical significance.

The intestinal variant of PanIN has a pseudostratified columnar epithelium with occasional goblet cells and dysplastic changes similar to those in colonic adenomas.[13] The intestinal variant was identified in association with colloid carcinoma (mucinous noncystic carcinoma).

The oncocytic variant of PanIN has cytoplasm that ranges from clear to eosinophilic/granular and large vesicular nuclei with prominent nucleoli.[13] The oncocytic variant may also have dystrophic goblet cells.

Recently, a foamy gland variant of PanIN has been described.[14] This variant was found in association with the foamy gland variant of invasive ductal adenocarcinoma. The PanIN-1 lesions associated with invasive foamy gland carcinomas were indistinguishable from conventional PanIN-1 lesions. The PanIN-2 and PanIN-3 lesions, however, had a unique morphology with mixtures of foamy cells and conventional dysplastic cells and occasional dilation of small ducts.[14]

LOBULOCENTRIC ATROPHY AND ACINAR DUCTAL METAPLASIA

Lobulocentric atrophy is the progressive atrophy of a single lobule and is frequently found in

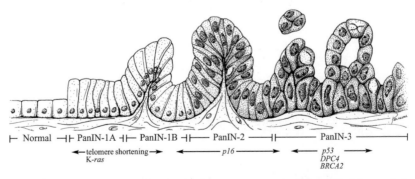

Fig. 2. PanIN grading. PanINs are graded morphologically along a continuum of increasingly dysplastic features. Molecular studies have confirmed that this grading system parallels a stepwise accumulation of genetic abnormalities commonly found in invasive ductal adenocarcinoma. Telomere shortening and KRAS mutations are early changes that can be found in low-grade lesions. p16 inactivation is a later event commonly found in intermediate lesions, whereas BRCA2, TP53, and DPC4/SMAD4 inactivation is common only in PanIN-3 and invasive ductal adenocarcinoma. (*From* Wilentz RE, Iacobuzio-Donahue CA, Argani P, et al. Loss of expression of Dpc4 in pancreatic intraepithelial neoplasia: evidence that DPC4 inactivation occurs late in neoplastic progression. Cancer Res 2000;60:2005; with permission.)

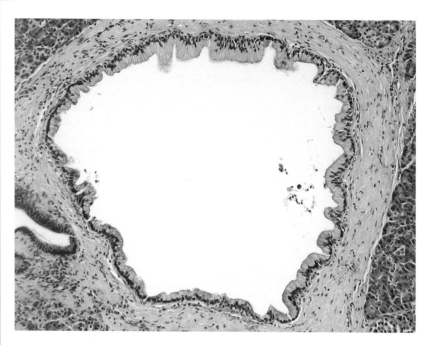

Fig. 3. PanIN, grade 1A. PanIN-1A has a predominantly flat columnar epithelium with abundant supranuclear mucin and basally oriented, round nuclei. Dysplasia is not striking.

association with a PanINs.[15,16] This association is seen in patients with sporadic pancreatic cancer as well as in patients with a significant family history of pancreatic cancer.[15–17]

Lobulocentric atrophy resembles a focal version of the widespread change that occurs after ligation of the pancreatic duct (**Fig. 7**). In lobulocentric atrophy, some acinar cells are lost whereas others seem to undergo acinar ductal metaplasia (ADM). In ADM, acinar cells lose their granules and flatten to form a thin duct-like epithelium (**Fig. 8**).[15] The lumen may subsequently dilate and the cells blend almost imperceptibly into a PanIN morphology.[16] Inflammation and progressive fibrosis accompany this process, and eventually only the islet cells remain.

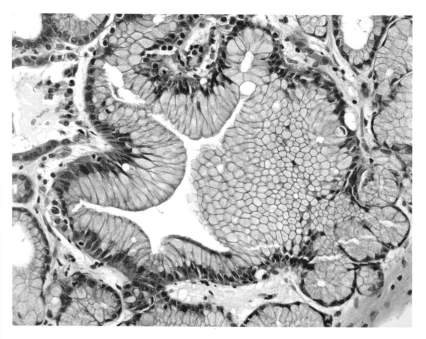

Fig. 4. PanIN, grade 1B. PanIN-1B has similar cytologic features to PanIN-1A but has a more pronounced papillary or micropapillary architecture.

Fig. 5. PanIN, grade 2. PanIN-2 typically has a prominent papillary architecture and mild-to-moderate cytologic atypia, including hyperchromasia, increased nuclear size, crowding, pseudostratification, and some loss of polarity.

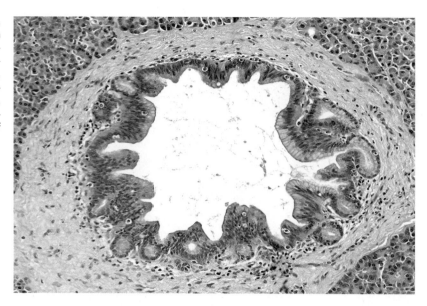

The underlying mechanism for ADM and its association with PanIN is not clear. Animal models of pancreatic cancer are associated with ADM lesions leading to the hypothesis that the acinar cell, through ADM, is the cell of origin for invasive ductal adenocarcinoma in these models.[18–22] Recent analysis of KRAS2 mutations in human ADMs suggests, however, that the PanIN forms first, causing a local duct obstruction that induces lobulocentric atrophy and secondary ADM formation.[23] The resulting epithelial injury and fibrosis may then promote dysplastic progression of the PanIN lesion.[16] The sequence of these events remains speculative until the temporal and microanatomic relationships between PanINs, ADMs, and lobulocentric atrophy are better defined.

Fig. 6. PanIN, grade 3. PanIN-3 has marked nuclear and cytologic atypia but lacks an invasive component. These lesions have a papillary, micropapillary, or cribriform architecture and widespread loss of nuclear polarity. Mitoses, including occasional abnormal mitoses, are seen.

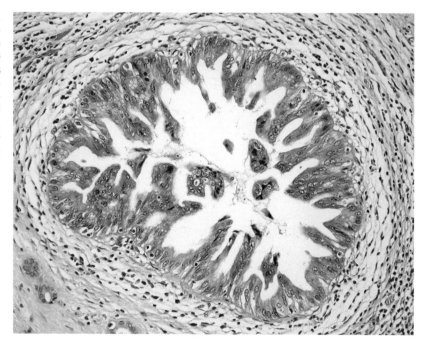

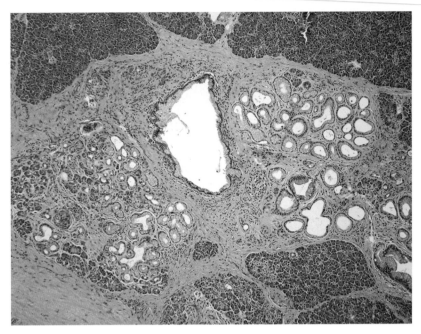

Fig. 7. Lobulocentric atrophy and associated PanIN. An area of lobulocentric atrophy is flanked by uninvolved pancreas. Chronic inflammation and fibrosis infiltrate the lobule and few acini remain intact. Low-grade PanIN is present in the central, larger duct and throughout the atrophic lobule in a pattern typical of lobulocentric atrophy.

IMMUNOPHENOTYPE

PanINs, IPMNs, and invasive ductal adenocarcinomas have distinct mucin immunophenotypes for MUC1 (panepithelial surface mucin), MUC2 (intestinal-type mucin), and MUC5AC (gastric foveolar-type mucin). Invasive ductal adenocarcinoma strongly expresses MUC1 and MUC5AC and is negative for MUC2.[24] PanINs, especially high-grade PanINs, display an immunophenotype similar to that of invasive ductal adenocarcinoma.[25] MUC5AC and MUC6 (gastric pyloric-type mucin) are expressed by all grades of PanIN, whereas MUC1 is most consistently expressed in higher-grade lesions.[26] PanINs with a conventional morphology are almost always negative for

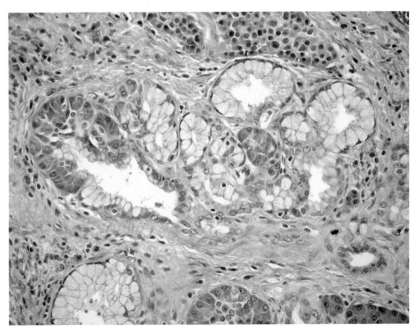

Fig. 8. Acinar ductal metaplasia. Pancreatic acini can undergo a progressive metaplasia, developing a dilated lumen with a flattened cuboidal lining. Frequently, areas of ADM are intimately associated with mucinous columnar epithelium typical of PanIN.

MUC2.[25] In contrast, intestinal-type IPMNs are usually negative for MUC1 and frequently express MUC2.[25]

The rare foamy gland variant of PanIN has an immunophenotype identical to conventional PanIN.[14] In contrast, the oncocytic variant of PanIN is positive for both MUC1 and MUC2, whereas the intestinal variant is negative for MUC1 and positive for MUC2.[13]

MOLECULAR FEATURES

The progressive dysplasia in PanINs is mirrored by an accumulation of genetic alterations also found in invasive pancreatic adenocarcinoma. Telomere length, shortening is associated with chromosomal instability. This seems to be an early event in carcinogenesis because telomeres are significantly shorter in the vast majority of PanINs, including 91% of PanIN-1A lesions.[27] Mutations of the KRAS oncogene are also common in pancreatic ductal adenocarcinoma, and these mutations are found in approximately one-third of PanIN-1A lesions, close to half of PanIN-1B lesions, and more than three-fourths of PanIN-2/3 lesions associated with invasive carcinoma.[9,28–31] A similar progression is observed with the tumor suppressor gene, p16INK4A/CDKN2A. p16 is frequently inactivated in pancreatic adenocarcinoma and shows a loss of expression in 30% of PanIN-1A/B, 55% of PanIN-2, and 71% of PanIN-3 lesions associated with carcinoma.[6,32]

Other tumor suppressor genes are lost late in pancreatic carcinogenesis: both TP53 and DPC4/SMAD4 are commonly inactivated in invasive pancreatic adenocarcinoma, and these genes are only inactivated in advanced PanIN-3 lesions.[6,32] Several other genetic changes display a similar progression.[33]

Recently it was demonstrated that microRNAs known to be overexpressed in pancreatic adenocarcinoma are also overexpressed in high-grade PanIN. A significant increase in miR-155 is observed in PanIN-2 with a greater increase in PanIN-3.[34] Overexpression of miR-21 has also been confirmed as an early event in PanIN formation, with increased expression in higher-grade PanINs.[34,35]

DIFFERENTIAL DIAGNOSIS

INVASIVE DUCTAL ADENOCARCINOMA

Invasive well-differentiated ductal adenocarcinoma is by far the most important entity in the differential diagnosis of PanIN lesions. Well-differentiated invasive ductal adenocarcinoma can often be bland, making well-formed glands with minimal cytologic atypia. In isolation, these well-differentiated carcinomas can closely resemble low-grade PanIN lesions and present a significant diagnostic challenge, especially on frozen sections. Less commonly, a moderately differentiated invasive carcinoma can mimic a higher-grade PanIN (**Fig. 9**). In these cases,

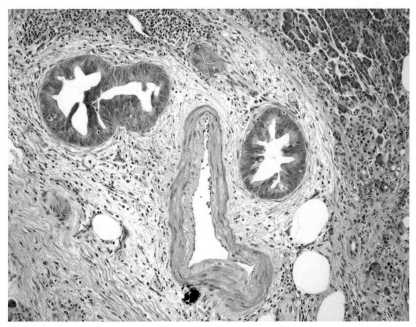

Fig. 9. Invasive ductal adenocarcinoma mimicking PanIN-3. Two foci of invasive ductal adenocarcinoma display architecture and cytology consistent with PanIN-3; however, their close proximity to a medium-sized vessel is a helpful clue to their true nature.

Differential Diagnosis
PanIN

- Invasive ductal adenocarcinoma
  - Invasive ductal adenocarcinoma can display minimal cytologic atypia that falls short of established diagnostic criteria.
  - PanINs should display a normal lobular architecture, whereas an invasive ductal adenocarcinoma shows a haphazard growth pattern.
  - Invasion of vessels or nerves is almost exclusively a feature of invasive carcinoma.
  - A gland immediately adjacent to a muscular vessel is highly suggestive of invasive adenocarcinoma.
- Cancerization of benign pancreatic ducts
  - An abrupt transition between normal duct (or a low-grade PanIN) to highly dysplastic epithelium is typical of cancerization.
  - An invasive ductal adenocarcinoma nearby should raise suspicion.
- Vascular invasion with extension along vascular lumen
  - The presence of a vessel wall may be subtle, but the location is usually not part of the normal lobular architecture.
  - Special stains can confirm the presence of a surrounding vessel.
- Intraductal papillary mucinous neoplasm
  - IPMNs are usually grossly identifiable as cysts.
  - IPMNs measure greater than 1.0 cm whereas PanINs are less than 0.5 cm.
  - PanINs tend to have shorter, less complex papillary structures than IPMNs.
  - Intermediate lesions (0.5 to 1.0 cm) may be considered incipient IPMNs.
  - Expression of MUC2 suggests an intestinal type IPMN.
- Reactive epithelial changes
  - Nuclear atypia tends to be less severe than in PanIN.
  - Hesitate before making the diagnosis of PanIN in the presence of acute inflammation.
- Squamous metaplasia
  - Mature squamous epithelium replaces the glandular ductal epithelium.
  - This should not be mistaken for an area of high-grade dysplasia.

identifying the pattern of growth is critical to making a confident diagnosis. Do the glands in question conform to the lobular branching pattern of the normal pancreas, or are they haphazardly arranged and in areas of the pancreas where benign glands are usually not seen? Even in the presence of significant fibrosis, PanINs maintain a typical lobular architecture whereas invasive cancers do not. Intimate association of glandular structures with nerves is virtually diagnostic of invasive carcinoma. Because non-neoplastic pancreatic ducts are almost always separated from muscular vessels

by pancreatic parenchyma, several groups have found the presence of a gland in immediate proximity to a muscular vessel a helpful feature in identifying a gland as belonging to an invasive adenocarcinoma.[36]

CANCERIZATION OF BENIGN PANCREATIC DUCTS

Invasive ductal adenocarcinoma can invade benign ducts or ductules (or even low-grade PanINs) and grow along the luminal surface displacing the epithelium and mimicking a high grade PanIN.

Hallmarks of cancerization are similar to those found in other sites. An abrupt, stair-step transition from an entirely benign, non-neoplastic epithelium to a highly dysplastic-appearing epithelium is suspicious for cancerization. Close proximity of a PanIN to an invasive ductal adenocarcinoma in the adjacent stroma should also raise suspicion. If the distinction between PanIN-3 and invasive ductal adenocarcinoma becomes clinically relevant, serial sections can sometimes uncover a direct connection to an obviously invasive focus.

VASCULAR INVASION WITH INTRAVASCULAR EXTENSION

When ductal adenocarcinoma has invaded the vasculature, it is not uncommon for the cancer to extend along the luminal surface of the vessel. When invasive carcinoma involves the vessel in this manner, the vessel can closely mimic the appearance of a PanIN. This is especially true when the vascular invasion has a very low-grade appearance and closely resembles a PanIN-1 lesion (**Fig. 10**A). The location

Fig. 10. Vascular invasion mimicking PanIN-1. Invasive ductal adenocarcinoma in a vessel grows along the luminal surface, creating the appearance of low-grade PanIN. (*A*) Mucinous epithelium is clearly visible in the hematoxylin-eosin stained section. (*B*) The epithelium is mostly lost on a corresponding Verhoeff-van Gieson stain, but the stain highlights the elastic fibers present in the vessel wall.

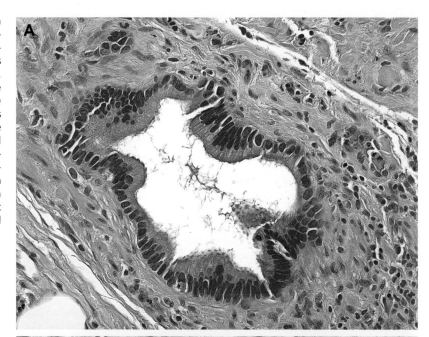

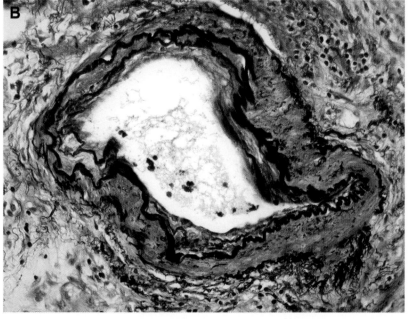

of the lesion can be helpful because vessels do not typically conform to a lobular structure. A Verhoeff-van Gieson stain or other stain that highlights vessels can be helpful in uncertain cases (see **Fig. 10B**).

INTRADUCTAL PAPILLARY MUCINOUS NEOPLASM

The distinction between a large PanIN and a small IPMN is somewhat arbitrary. PanINs tend to have papillary structures that are shorter and less complex than the long, almost finger-like papillae of IPMNs. In general, the authors consider lesions less than 0.5 cm in greatest dimension to be Pan-INs and those lesions measuring greater than 1.0 cm to be IPMNs. Lesions of intermediate size (between 0.5 and 1.0 cm) may be classified as incipient IPMNs.[23] Mucin immunophenotyping may also be used to distinguish ambiguous lesions.[26] The expression of MUC2 suggests an intestinal-type IPMN.

REACTIVE EPITHELIAL CHANGES

Reactive epithelial changes manifest predominantly with nuclear enlargement, hyperchromasia, and prominent nucleoli. Caution should be exercised when diagnosing dysplasia in the presence of acute inflammation. Distinguishing reactive changes from true dysplasia is usually not difficult because reactive changes tend to lack the architectural features of PanINs. Reactive nuclei also tend to have smooth contours, finely distributed chromatin, and abundant cytoplasm.

SQUAMOUS METAPLASIA

Replacement of the ductal epithelium by mature squamous epithelium is a relatively common benign finding in pancreatic resections (**Fig. 11**). Squamous metaplasia is most likely the product of repeated duct injury and is commonly associated with calculi. Nuclear atypia is generally not present in foci of squamous metaplasia, and it should not be mistaken for high-grade PanIN.

DIAGNOSIS

Because the pancreas is infrequently biopsied, the diagnosis of PanIN is made almost exclusively in specimens resected for other reasons. The diagnosis and grading of PanINs are primarily based on the morphology of the lesion but also informed by the greatest dimension of the lesion, which should generally be less than 0.5 cm. When reporting the presence of PanIN, only the highest grade of PanIN needs to be reported. As discussed later, great caution should be exerted in reporting the presence of high-grade PanIN at a resection margin because it is all too easy for clinicians to overreact to a PanIN at a margin and to overtreat a patient for a lesion of unproved clinical significance.

Unlike the macroscopic pancreatic cancer precursors (MCN and IPMN), in vivo imaging does

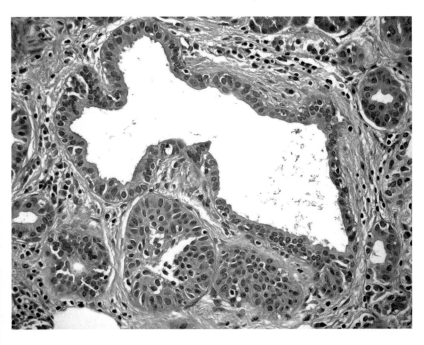

Fig. 11. Squamous metaplasia. Pancreatic ducts and ductules frequently undergo squamous metaplasia but these foci should not be mistaken for a high-grade PanIN.

not currently play a significant role in the detection or diagnosis of PanINs. Clinically, no imaging technique can directly detect PanINs, although there is a clear need for such a technique to detect and monitor PanINs in high-risk patients. Endoscopic ultrasound is the best available method for detecting PanINs in vivo, although this method indirectly images PanINs by detecting the fibrosis in the multifocal PanIN-associated lobulocentric atrophy commonly found in high-risk patients.[16] Endoscopic ultrasound has been used in screening individuals with a strong family history of pancreatic cancer (2 or more first-degree relatives) and this screening technique is used in an ongoing multicenter study.[37]

PROGNOSIS

POTENTIAL FOR PROGRESSION TO INVASIVE CARCINOMA

Although PanIN is a precursor to invasive ductal adenocarcinoma, the rate of progression from low-grade PanIN to invasive carcinoma is low and has been estimated to be less than 1%.[9] Direct evidence of this progression is lacking primarily because there are no adequate surveillance methods to follow the natural progression of PanIN. Indirect evidence of progression comes from several reports of patients who had partial pancreatectomies.[38,39] PanIN-3 was identified in these 4 reported cases. In 3 of these cases, PanIN-3 extended to the resection margin, whereas in the fourth it was extensive and multifocal. These patients subsequently presented with invasive ductal adenocarcinoma of the remaining pancreas after intervals of 17 months, 9 years, 10 years, and 29 years, strongly suggesting that high-grade PanIN present in the residual pancreas progressed to invasive carcinoma.[38,39] As discussed previously, molecular genetic analyses of PanIN lesions and genetically engineered mouse models probably provide the strongest evidence linking PanINs to invasive adenocarcinoma.

SIGNIFICANCE OF PanIN AT A SURGICAL MARGIN

The presence of PanIN at a surgical margin is of uncertain significance. The cases (discussed previously) provide some evidence that invasive carcinoma may develop after a pancreatectomy with a PanIN-3 positive margin.[38,39] In practice, the authors report the presence of high-grade PanIN-3 when it is present at a resection margin but recommend resecting additional tissue only when the PanIN is extensive and a patient's clinical context suggests it could be of prognostic significance. For example, a PanIN-3 lesion present at the pancreatic neck margin in an 80-year-old man with a 5-cm invasive pancreatic adenocarcinoma and lymph node metastases is insignificant. By contrast, extensive PanIN-3 lesions at the margin of a 25-year-old patient with a small well-differentiated pancreatic endocrine neoplasm may justify the resection of additional pancreatic parenchyma. Surgical pathologists must communicate with their surgeons and be familiar with a surgeon's understanding of the lesion and the action it will elicit. Extensive additional resection to chase PanINs is usually unwarranted.

REFERENCES

1. Surveillance epidemiology and end results: SEER stat facts sheets, pancreatic cancer. Available at: http://seer.cancer.gov/statfacts/html/pancreas.html. Accessed July 1, 2009.
2. Klimstra DS, Longnecker DS. K-ras mutations in pancreatic ductal proliferative lesions. Am J Pathol 1994;145(6):1547–50.
3. Hruban RH, Takaori K, Klimstra DS, et al. An illustrated consensus on the classification of pancreatic intraepithelial neoplasia and intraductal papillary mucinous neoplasms. Am J Surg Pathol 2004; 28(8):977–87.
4. Hruban RH, Adsay NV, Albores-Saavedra J, et al. Pancreatic intraepithelial neoplasia: a new nomenclature and classification system for pancreatic duct lesions. Am J Surg Pathol 2001;25(5):579–86.
5. Andea A, Sarkar F, Adsay VN. Clinicopathological correlates of pancreatic intraepithelial neoplasia: a comparative analysis of 82 cases with and 152 cases without pancreatic ductal adenocarcinoma. Mod Pathol 2003;16(10):996–1006.
6. Moskaluk CA, Hruban RH, Kern SE. p16 and K-ras gene mutations in the intraductal precursors of human pancreatic adenocarcinoma. Cancer Res 1997;57(11):2140–3.
7. Kozuka S, Sassa R, Taki T, et al. Relation of pancreatic duct hyperplasia to carcinoma. Cancer 1979; 43(4):1418–28.
8. Pour PM, Sayed S, Sayed G. Hyperplastic, preneoplastic and neoplastic lesions found in 83 human pancreases. Am J Clin Pathol 1982;77(2):137–52.
9. Terhune PG, Phifer DM, Tosteson TD, et al. K-ras mutation in focal proliferative lesions of human pancreas. Cancer Epidemiol Biomarkers Prev 1998;7(6):515–21.
10. Shi C, Klein AP, Goggins M, et al. Increased prevalence of precursor lesions in familial pancreatic cancer patients. Clin Cancer Res 2009;15(24):7737–43.
11. Rebours V, Levy P, Mosnier JF, et al. Pathology analysis reveals that dysplastic pancreatic ductal

using endoscopic ultrasonography fine-needle aspiration. Mucin-secreting cells or elevated tumor markers with high levels of carcinoembryonic antigen (CEA, >400 ng/mL) and carbohydrate antigen (CA) 19.9 (>50,000 U/mL) are strongly suggestive of mucinous neoplasms.[5] In contrast to pseudocysts, cyst amylase levels are usually normal in MCNs; however, preoperative diagnosis of MCNs remains difficult both on imaging and on cytology. A major pitfall for the latter is gastrointestinal epithelial contamination, which can lead to a misdiagnosis of mucinous tumors.

MACROSCOPIC FEATURES

The MCNs present as large, round cystic masses (average size of 6 to 10 cm) with a unilocular or multilocular cut surface (**Fig. 1**). Papillary projections and mural nodules can be observed and correspond frequently with areas of malignancy.[10] The tumors are usually filled with an abundant clear mucoid fluid. The wall of the cyst may be dense and fibrous with occasionally foci of calcification and can be confused with a pseudocyst.

MICROSCOPIC FEATURES

MCNs are characterized by 2 distinct histologic components: (1) an inner epithelial layer composed of tall mucin-secreting cells and (2) a dense cellular ovarian-type stroma. The latter, which is now required for the diagnosis of MCN, forms a band of densely packed spindle-shaped cells immediately beneath the neoplastic epithelium (**Fig. 2**). These spindle-shaped cells can even show luteinization with clusters of epithelioid cells (**Fig. 3**). Presence of such stroma can be helpful for diagnosis, particularly when the epithelial lining is extensively denuded (**Fig. 4**); however, it can be partially or even completely hyalinized and

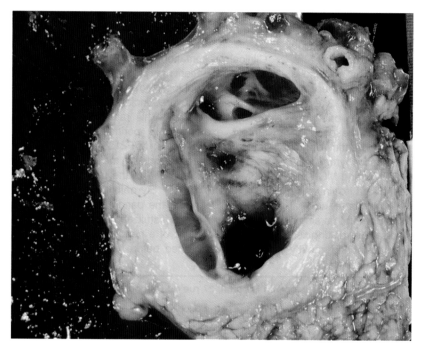

Fig. 1. Macroscopic view of MCN occurring in the tail of the pancreas. This multilocular cystic lesion is separated by thin septations and surrounded by a thick capsule.

Fig. 2. MCN with low-grade dysplasia. Note the ovarian-type stroma immediately beneath the epithelium lining (hematoxylin-esoin [H&E] stain, original magnification ×20).

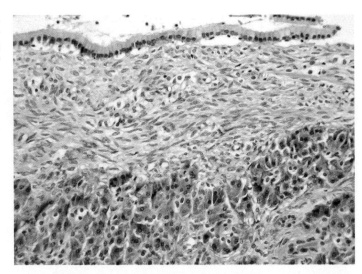

Fig. 3. MCN showing in the ovarian-type stroma the presence of luteinized cells with eosinophilic cytoplasm (hematoxylin phloxine saffron [HPS] stain, original magnification ×10).

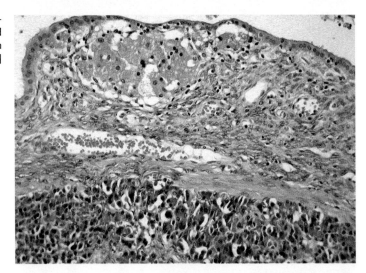

Fig. 4. MCN revealing extensive denudation of the epithelial lining. Characterization of the ovarian-type stroma is helpful for the diagnosis (HPS stain, original magnification ×10).

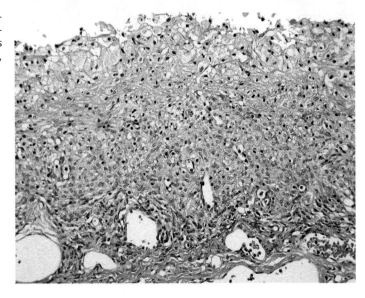

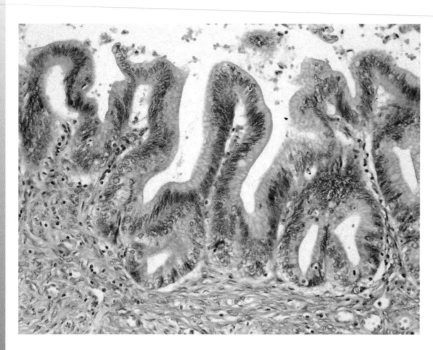

Fig. 5. MCN with intermediate-grade dysplasia (H&E stain, original magnification ×20).

extensive sampling is needed.[10] Inversely, there can be a predominant overgrowing epithelial component, creating a solid tumor.[13] Sarcomatous transformation of this ovarian-type stroma has been reported in rare cases.[14]

The epithelial component consists of columnar mucin-producing cells with various degrees of architectural and nuclear atypia (see **Fig. 1**; **Figs. 5** and **6**).[11] The epithelium can be flat or papillary, and epithelium with significant dysplasia is often immediately adjacent to entirely benign epithelium. The columnar epithelium stains with periodic acid-Schiff in most cases and with Alcian blue in about 66% of cases. This staining may be

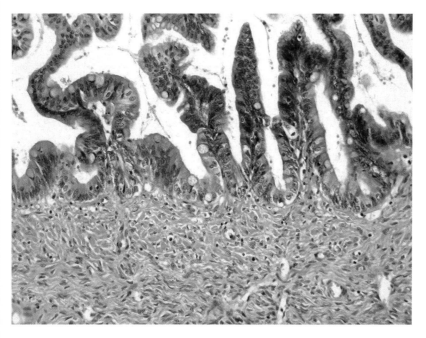

Fig. 6. MCN with high-grade dysplasia (H&E stain, original magnification ×20).

confined to the apical border of the cells. Goblet cells, endocrine cells, and Paneth cells may also be found in the epithelium (**Fig. 7**). Adequate sampling of MCN is important to properly evaluate these neoplasms. The chance of finding dysplastic or invasive foci is greater in the thickened fibrotic walls and septae, as well as in intramural nodules projecting into the cyst lumen. According to the architectural complexity and cytologic atypia, noninvasive MCNs are sub-classified into MCNs with low-grade dysplasia, intermediate-grade dysplasia, and high-grade dysplasia.[15] In MCNs with low-grade dysplasia, the lining epithelium is usually flat and exhibits minimal or mild cytologic atypia (see **Fig. 2**). MCNs with intermediate-grade dysplasia show papillary projections and nuclear stratification (see **Fig. 5**). MCNs with high-grade dysplasia are characterized by irregular branching papillae or cribriform structures with severe cytologic atypia (see **Fig. 6**).

An invasive carcinoma is present in fewer than one-third of MCNs (**Fig. 8**).[7,9] It can be focal and confined to the wall of the cyst or extend into the surrounding pancreatic tissue or adjacent organs; however, lymph node metastases are rare or absent.[9] The invasive foci are usually of tubular/ductal type but other rare variants have been described, such as adenosquamous carcinoma and undifferentiated carcinoma with or without osteoclast giant cells.[16,17] In contrast, pure colloid carcinoma, which is frequently observed in IPMNs, is extremely rare in MCNs.

IMMUNOHISTOCHEMISTRY

Morphology remains the mainstay for the diagnosis of MCN. When immunohistochemistry is used, the epithelium lining the cysts is immunoreactive with cytokeratins 7, 8, 18, 19, and 20; CD10; CEA; and gastric-type mucin marker MUC5AC.[11,18,19] Scattered gobletlike cells express the intestinal mucin marker MUC2. As in ductal adenocarcinomas, the invasive component of MCNs may acquire the expression of MUC1, which is not usually expressed in noninvasive forms.[20] Similarly, expression of DPC4 is frequently lost in the invasive component.[21] The ovarian-type stroma expresses progesterone receptors and estrogen receptors in 70% and 30% of cases respectively. Luteinized cells included in this stroma are positive for calretinin, alpha-inhibin, and tyrosine hydroxylase (**Fig. 9**).[10,19]

PATHOGENESIS

Although pancreatic MCNs show similar pathologic features with their counterparts in the hepatobiliary tract, the ovary, or the retroperitoneum, their origin remains largely unknown. Two hypotheses have been formulated to explain such neoplasms associated with an ovarian-type stroma. The first hypothesis is that these neoplasms arise from an ectopic ovarian stroma. This is supported by the close proximity of the left primordial gonad to the dorsal pancreas during the fifth week of gestation, possibly facilitating the transfer of cells.[22] Of course, such a hypothesis

Fig. 7. MCN showing goblet cells in the lining epithelium (H&E stain, original magnification ×10).

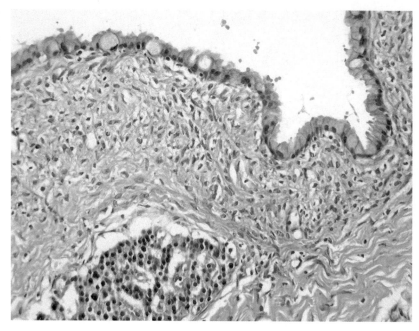

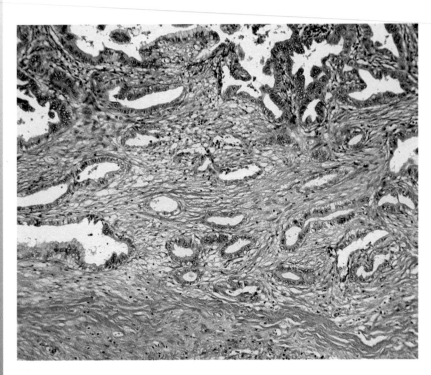

Fig. 8. MCN with a foci of tubular adenocarcinoma infiltrating the wall of the cyst (HPS stain, original magnification ×5).

cannot account for rare MCNs arising in males. The second hypothesis is that the ovarian-type stroma represents an equivalent of periductal fetal mesenchyme, the primitive mesenchyme seen around the pancreatic and hepatic ducts in the developing fetus.[23] This last hypothesis could similarly explain mucinous cystadenoma occurring in the hepatobiliary tract. Regardless of its origin, it is clear that female sex hormones might have had a role in the pathogenesis of this neoplasm.

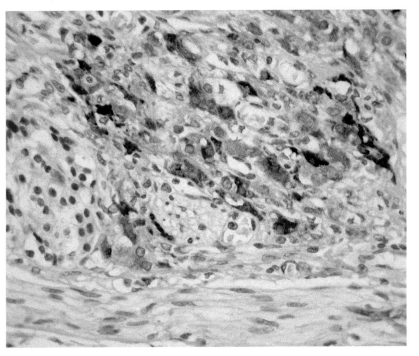

Fig. 9. MCN containing a cluster of luteinized cells positive for alpha-inhibin (immunohistochemistry, original magnification ×40).

This stroma is hormone sensitive and luteinized cells, which are present in 40% of cases, are capable of steroidogenesis.

DIFFERENTIAL DIAGNOSIS

A difficult differential diagnosis can be raised with a pseudocyst, as large areas of denudation of the epithelial lining and fibrosis involvement of ovarian-type stroma may occur in MCNs.[10] In such cases, extensive sampling to identify well-preserved areas is often needed. Other differential diagnoses of MCNs include retention cysts with mucinous metaplastic features, IPMNs, and serous cystic neoplasms. The non-neoplastic retention cyst corresponds to a single unilocular cyst, which is lined by mucin-producing cells without atypia. It occurs mainly in the head of the pancreas. The pancreatic parenchyma closed to the dilated duct shows fibrosis and lobular atrophy. MCNs also must be distinguished from IPMNs (**Table 1**), particularly those involving the branch ducts. As seen in following sections, these 2 entities exhibit different pathologic features and biologic behavior, including prevalence of invasive cancer and recurrence rate after radical resection. In contrast to MCNs, IPMNs involve the pancreatic duct and do not contain the ovarian-type stroma. Because this latter histologic criterion is now required in the current definition of MCN, the proportion of MCNs relative to IPMNs is declining in most series. Serous cystic neoplasms, in particular the oligocystic variant, can be distinguished from MCNs by the presence of clear cuboidal cells lining some microcysts located in the wall of the tumor.[23] Other cystic neoplasms, such as solid-pseudopapillary neoplasms and cystic endocrine neoplasms, are easily distinguished because of the lack of mucin-producing columnar epithelium.

PROGNOSIS

In contrast to ordinary ductal adenocarcinoma, MCNs show an often-indolent biologic behavior, highlighting the importance of distinguishing these 2 entities.[9,24] However, until recently, discordant data concerning the prognosis existed because ovarian-type stroma was not defined in several series as a diagnostic criterion for MCNs.[7,8,25] Thus, IPMNs, especially of branch duct type, were probably integrated in some previous studies. In a recent large series of 163 "pure" MCNs,[9] the 5-year disease-specific survival was 100% and 57% for those without and with invasive carcinomas respectively. Prevalence of invasive carcinoma was only 12% and highly correlated with the size of the neoplasms (>40 mm). Accurate prognosis of MCNs depends of the presence and the extent of an invasive component, as noninvasive lesions follow a benign course with no recurrence after surgical resection. In invasive forms, it is important to evaluate the depth of invasion, as the prognosis appears worse for neoplasms showing a peritumoral invasion than those limited to the cyst wall.[10]

INTRADUCTAL PAPILLARY MUCINOUS NEOPLASMS

OVERVIEW

Intraductal papillary mucinous neoplasms (IPMNs) are the most frequent cystic mucinous tumors occurring in the pancreas. They account for about 7% of clinically diagnosed pancreatic neoplasms and represent the second indication for pancreatic resection in referral centers after ductal adenocarcinoma.[5] IPMNs correspond to a grossly visible (typically >1 cm) intraductal proliferation of neoplastic mucin-producing cells involving the main pancreatic duct and/or its major branches predominantly in the head of the pancreas (70% to 80%). Both the variability of the location of these lesions and the severity of the disease is probably at the origin of the numerous appellations given to IPMNs in the past, such as main duct ectasia, branch duct xectasia, intraductal adenoma, papillomatosis, and mucus-secreting tumor.[26–28] IPMNs occur in men slightly more frequently than in women (male:female ratio of 60:40), and the median age at diagnosis is 66 years. Presenting signs and symptoms include long history of

---

△△ **Differential Diagnosis**
OF MUCINOUS CYSTIC
NEOPLASMS

1. Pseudocysts: MCNs with extensive epithelial denudation and fibrotic involution of the ovarian-type stroma need to be differentiated from pseudocysts. Extensive sampling to identify well-preserved areas of MCNs is required.

2. Branch duct-type IPMN: MCNs show an ovarian-type stroma and are not communicated with the ductal system.

3. Other cystic neoplasms: In contrast to MCNs, no mucinous epithelial lining is observed.

Table 1
Differential diagnosis of mucinous cystic neoplasms and intraductal papillary mucinous neoplasms

Features	Mucinous Cystic Neoplasms	Intraductal Papillary Mucinous Neoplasms
Age, median, y	45	66
Female, %	95%	30%–40%
Location	Body-tail (96%)	Head (>80%)
Specific endoscopic finding	None	Mucin extrusion from ampulla
Communication with ductal system	No	Yes
Presence of ovarian stroma	Yes	No
Rate of invasive carcinoma, %	12%	30%

epigastric pain, weight loss, steatorrhea, and recurrent pancreatitis with ductal dilatation.[29–32] These symptoms are caused by intermittent obstruction of the ductal system by globs of mucin. Increasingly, IPMNs are incidentally detected by imaging, particularly those confined to the branch ducts.[5] Depending of the part of the pancreatic duct system involved, computed tomography, magnetic resonance imaging, and endoscopic ultrasonography abdominal imaging reveal either a diffuse dilatation of the main duct and its branch ducts or a more circumscribed cystic lesion developed from rare branch ducts. The diagnosis of IPMNs can be highly suspected when mucus extruding from the ampulla is visualized. As in MCNs, mucin atypical cells and elevated tumor markers (CEA, CA 19.9, and CA 72.4) in cyst fluid may aid in establishing the diagnosis of mucinous tumors.

Key Points
INTRADUCTAL PAPILLARY MUCINOUS NEOPLASMS (IPMNs)

1. IPMNs are intraductal proliferations of neoplastic mucin-producing cells involving the main pancreatic duct and/or its major branches predominantly in the head of the pancreas.

2. They are frequently detected incidentally and constitute a heterogeneous group with at least 4 subtypes (intestinal, gastric, pancreaticobiliary, and oncocytic).

3. IPMNs of branch duct type show a more indolent course than the main duct type.

4. Like MCNs, the prognosis is correlated with the presence of an invasive component.

MACROSCOPIC FEATURES

Most IPMNs arise in the head or uncinate process of the pancreas (75%); however, IPMNs can also arise in the body or tail of the gland (20%), and rare IPMNs diffusely involve the entire length of the pancreas.[33] Macroscopically, the pancreas shows a cystic dilatation of the ductal system, an intraductal proliferation, and mucus accumulation. Extension and location of the intraductal proliferation is better defined after opening the pancreatic resection along the main duct. Depending on the location of the lesion in the main pancreatic duct or in the branch ducts, IPMN can be further subdivided into main duct and branch duct types respectively.

- In the main duct type, the main pancreatic duct is diffusely or focally dilated and contains abundant mucus secretion. Involvement of the branch ducts is frequently associated (**Fig. 10**). In florid cases, the intraductal proliferation is macroscopically detectable with endoluminal vegetation or mural nodules.[29] Any solid or firm areas should be sampled to rule out invasive adenocarcinoma. Although the neoplasm usually progresses in a continuous manner along the main pancreatic duct, extensive sampling permits identification of the rare multicentric IPMNs. The uninvolved pancreas often shows changes because of chronic obstruction.

- Macroscopic lesions in IPMN of branch duct type are typically smaller, less papillary, and less malignant. Most often, the involvement of branch ducts results in a circumscribed cystic lesion or a cluster of mildly dilated ducts (**Fig. 11**).[33] The rare cases of invasive carcinoma associated with branch duct type IPMN occur usually when the size of the cystic lesion is greater than 3 cm and/or mural nodules are present.[34–36] At distance of the cystic lesions, pancreas appears normal.

Fig. 10. Macroscopic appearance of IPMN exhibiting a major dilatation of the main duct and branch ducts.

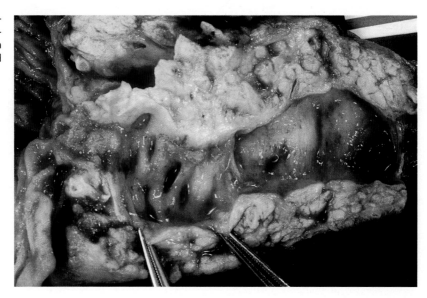

MICROSCOPIC FEATURES

Microscopically, the normal ductal epithelium is replaced by mucin-producing columnar cells showing papillary proliferations and variable degrees of cellular atypia (see **Fig. 11**). However, according to the differentiation of epithelial cells and the morphology of papillae, IPMNs form a group of heterogeneous neoplasms. They have been classified into 4 subtypes based on their histologic features and their mucin profiles[20,37–40]:

1. The intestinal type (50% of cases) appears similar to intestinal villous neoplasms with tall columnar epithelial cells showing a variable amount of apical mucin (**Fig. 12**). It occurs in the main pancreatic duct and the branch ducts and produces abundant mucin secretion.
2. The gastric type (40% of cases) exhibits small papillae lined by epithelial cells resembling gastric foveolar cells and shows pyloriclike glands at the base of the papillae (**Fig. 13**). Most of gastric-type IPMNs are benign and

Fig. 11. Branch duct type IPMN. The pancreatic branch duct shows a cystic dilatation and a florid papillary proliferation. Note that the main duct (on the *left*) is not involved in this proliferation (H&E stain, original magnification ×2.5).

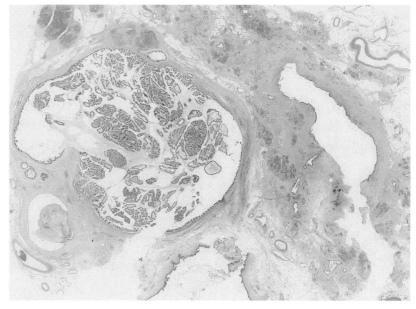

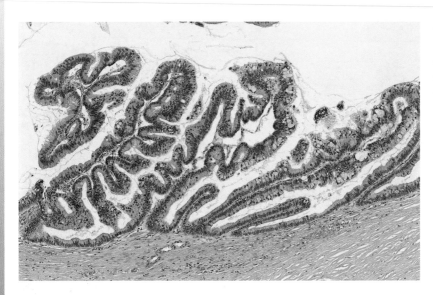

Fig. 12. Intestinal type of IPMN showing a villous growth pattern similar to that of villous adenoma of the colon (H&E stain, original magnification ×10).

reveal low-grade dysplasia. They involve the branch ducts forming benign multicystic lesions with cysts no larger than 3 cm.[41] In rare cases, the pyloric glands are prominent, forming polypoid masses in the lumen of the branch ducts. This form was previously called pyloric gland adenoma.

3. The pancreaticobiliary type (10% of cases) is composed of cuboidal cells resembling cholangiopapillary neoplasms (**Fig. 14**). It shows micropapillary structures with frequent high-grade dysplasia and an invasive component.

4. The oncocytic type (also called intraductal oncocytic papillary neoplasm) is the less common type.[42] It is composed of oncocytic cells forming polyps inside the lumen of the large ducts. It shows complex thick papillae lined by 2 to 5 layers of cuboidal cells with abundant eosinophilic granular cytoplasm (**Fig. 15**). Some scattered goblet cells can be

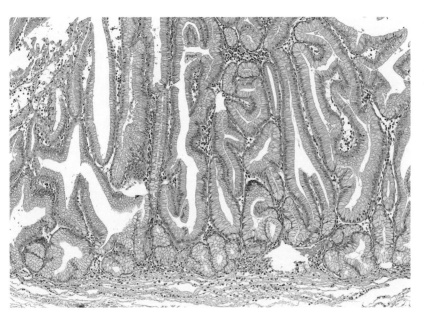

Fig. 13. Gastric type of IPMN exhibiting papillae lined by cells resembling gastric foveolar cells. Note the pyloric glandlike structures at the base of papillae (H&E stain, original magnification ×10).

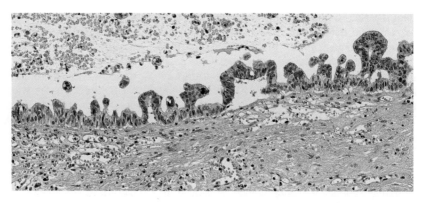

Fig. 14. Pancreaticobiliary type of IPMN showing micropapillae and severe cellular atypia (HPS stain, original magnification ×20).

seen. Most cases are classified as having high-grade dysplasia.

Most IPMNs, on the basis of the predominant architectural and cell-differentiation pattern, can be subclassified into one of these histologic subtypes; however, it is important to keep in mind that several directions of differentiation can be seen in individual IPMNs. In particular, a gastric type of epithelium may be seen together with intestinal or pancreaticobiliary types of epithelium.

All gradations according to the cytologic and architectural atypia of the proliferating epithelium may be encountered: IPMNs with low-grade dysplasia, intermediate-grade dysplasia, and high-grade dysplasia (carcinoma in situ).[15] The neoplasm is classified based on the highest, rather than the average, degree of atypia. IPMNs of low-grade dysplasia correspond mostly to gastric-type

IPMNs. Papillae are lined by a single layer of well-polarized cells showing minimal atypia. IPMN with intermediate-grade of dysplasia have nuclear hyperchromasia, nuclear crowding, and stratification. IPMNs of high-grade dysplasia are characterized by irregular projections lacking fibrovascular stalks. The nuclei show marked atypia and nuclear polarity is lost. An invasive component may be found in 30% to 40% of the cases. However, the prevalence of invasive cancer is highly variable according to the epithelial subtype of the IPMNs and the location of its involvement. Invasive carcinoma is frequently associated with the pancreaticobiliary type, whereas it is a rare event in the gastric type. Various reports have also demonstrated that there are significant differences in the presence of cancer between main duct IPMNs and branch duct IPMNs, ranging from 36% to 64% and 0% to 32%, respectively.[30,32,33,36,43] The fact that most branch

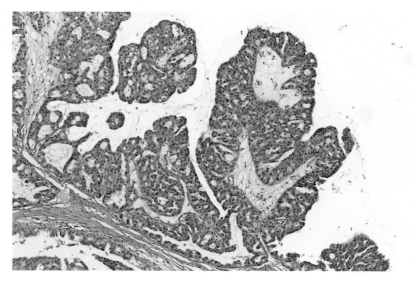

Fig. 15. Oncocytic type of IPMN characterized by complex arborizing papillae lined by oncocytic cells (H&E stain, original magnification ×5).

duct IPMNs are of the gastric type could partially explain such differences.[41] Two types of invasive adenocarcinoma arise in association with IPMNs.[39] Invasive colloid carcinoma is characterized by invasive large pools of extracellular mucin, occupying more than 80% of the tumoral surface, in which the neoplastic epithelial cells "float" (Fig. 16). It frequently arises in association with the intestinal type and must be distinguished from noninvasive IPMNs containing extraductal acellular mucin pools.[44] The second type of invasive adenocarcinoma associated with IPMNs is tubular adenocarcinoma, which is similar to ordinary ductal adenocarcinoma. This latter is frequently associated with pancreaticobiliary type.

IMMUNOHISTOCHEMISTRY

Like MCNs, IPMNs express different ductal markers including cytokeratins 7 and 19, CA19.9, and CEA. Mucin glycoproteins (MUCs) are useful markers for evaluating subtypes of IPMNs (Fig. 17). In normal pancreas, the interlobular ducts are negative for MUC1 and MUC2. The centroacinar cells and intralobular ducts, however, show consistent apical MUC1 staining. Overexpression of MUC1 is usually observed in conventional ductal adenocarcinoma. The intestinal type of IPMNs strongly express MUC2 and MUC5AC but not MUC1.[20,38,39] The intestinal differentiation of this subtype of IPMN is also underlined by the expression of CDX2. In contrast, the pancreaticobiliary type expresses MUC1 but not MUC2 or CDX2. The gastric type shows positivity for MUC5AC and for MUC6. The latter is usually expressed in the pyloriclike glands, which are associated with papillary proliferation. Not surprisingly, the mucin expression profile supports the existence of 2 different types of invasive tumor associated with IPMNs: colloid type is MUC2 positive and an ordinary ductal or tubular type is MUC1 positive. As mentioned previously, these carcinomas usually arise from intestinal-type and pancreaticobiliary-type IPMNs, respectively.[37,39] Other markers may underline the adenoma carcinoma progression with nuclear expression for TP53 and loss of expression for DPC4 and CDKN2A in IPMNs with invasive component or high-grade dysplasia.[21]

DIFFERENTIAL DIAGNOSIS

As we discussed previously, IPMNs need to be differentiated from MCNs. The latter affect women almost exclusively, occur predominantly in the pancreatic body or tail, do not communicate with the ductal system, and contain ovarian stroma. Differentiation of small IPMNs from pancreatic intraepithelial neoplasia (PanIN) lesions can be problematic, as both share many similar features. The separation of these 2 entities is based primarily on size.[45] Most PanINs are incidental microscopic findings that are not grossly or radiographically detectable, measuring smaller than 0.5 cm. By contrast, IPMNs are grossly identifiable, measuring typically more than 1.0 cm in size. Also, PanINs usually have gastric foveolar-type epithelium and do not express MUC2.[37] However, there are some cases, particularly cystic lesions measuring 0.5 to 1.0 cm, where such distinction can be virtually impossible. Because of these similarities, some investigators have formulated the hypothesis that

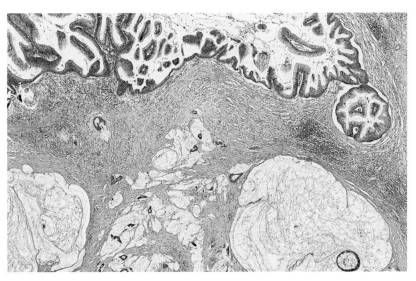

Fig. 16. Intestinal type of IPMN (upper) with colloid invasive carcinoma (lower). Note the presence of cluster of malignant cells within stromal pools of mucin (H&E stain, original magnification ×5).

	Pancreaticobiliary type	Intestinal type	Oncocytic type	Gastric type
IPMN				
MUC1				
MUC2				
MUC5AC				

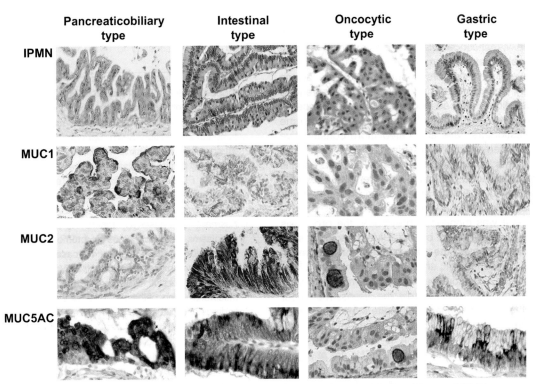

Fig. 17. Immunohistochemical profile of MUC1, MUC2, and MUC5AC expression in subtypes of IPMN.

IPMNs of the gastric type may arise from PanINs.[46] Retention cysts, unilocular cyst formations lined by flat mucinous ductal epithelium without atypia, must also be distinguished from IPMNs.[47]

IPMNs raise the differential diagnosis with other intraductal neoplasias, such as intraductal tubulopapillary neoplasms, intraductal acinar cell carcinomas, and rare cases of intraductal extension of primary ductal carcinomas, endocrine neoplasms, or metastasis (especially of a renal carcinoma). All of these entities usually reveal no mucin production. Intraductal tubulopapillary neoplasms show a complex glandular proliferation obliterating the ductal

lumen. The glands are lined by cuboidal cells showing high-grade dysplasia. The differential diagnosis is difficult, especially with IPMNs of pancreaticobiliary type.[48] The intraductal acinar cell carcinomas are highly cellular tumors composed of monotonous cellular populations arranged in acinar formations.[49,50] Illustration of enzyme production, such as trypsin, chymotrypsin, amylase, or lipase, by immunohistochemistry is necessary for diagnosis.

Microcystic serous adenomas have characteristic features that easily distinguish them from IPMNs. These neoplasms show a spongelike appearance and comprise numerous tiny cysts filled with serous fluid.[47] Often, the cysts are arranged around a central stellate scar. They are lined by cuboidal cells with clear cytoplasm. These neoplasms do not communicate with the pancreatic ductal system. The macrocystic serous variant, which can mimic the branch-duct IPMNs, shows the same clear and regular epithelium as that of the microcystic counterpart.[51]

Differential Diagnosis OF IPMNs

1. MCNs: IPMNs occur predominantly in the head of the pancreas, communicate with the ductal system, and do not show an ovarian-type stroma.

2. PanINs: These are microscopic lesions smaller than 5 mm.

3. Other rare intraductal neoplasias, such as intraductal tubulopapillary neoplasms.

TREATMENT AND PROGNOSIS

Currently, the only treatment of IPMN is surgical resection.[32,52,53] The extent of resection that is necessary is usually determined by histologic examination of the margins on frozen sections.[54] If

Key Features
SEROUS CYSTIC NEOPLASMS

1. Benign epithelial cystic neoplasm lined by bland cuboidal epithelial cells with clear cytoplasm and centrally located dark round nuclei

2. Most common serous cyst: Microcystic serous cystadenoma (composed of multiple small, cystic spaces) creating a characteristic honeycomb appearance on imaging studies and spongelike or grapefruitlike appearance on cut surface

3. Cyst fluid CEA levels should be low

4. Small, asymptomatic serous cysts may not need surgical intervention

Pitfalls
SEROUS CYSTIC NEOPLASMS

! The macrocystic variant (macrocystic serous cystadenoma) can mimic mucinous cysts or pseudocysts on imaging studies

! Fine-needle aspiration can cause cystic degeneration and partial denudation of the cyst lining, creating the appearance of a pseudocyst on the resected specimen

! A solid variant has been described

However, it appears that many more serous cystadenomas are being found incidentally, up to 50% in one study,[5] likely as the result of widespread use of imaging studies. Serous cystadenomas account for about 10% of surgically resected pancreatic cysts.[6,7] Because these cysts often do not produce symptoms, it is difficult to determine their true prevalence, but they have been reported to account for only 1% to 2% of all pancreatic exocrine neoplasms.[7,8]

Pancreatic cysts, typically serous cystadenomas or congenital cysts, occur in 30% to 72% of patients with von Hippel-Lindau (VHL) disease and may be the first manifestation of the disease.[9–12] In VHL disease, the pancreatic cysts typically do not produce symptoms, are discovered at a younger age (mean, 37 years), are often macrocystic, and may be multiple/diffuse.[12,13] Histologically, these cysts are identical to nonsyndromic cysts. Because of this macrocystic appearance and occurrence in younger patients, serous cystadenomas, in at least some reports, may represent the "congenital pancreatic cysts" seen in patients with VHL.

Two major variants of serous cystadenoma exist, microcystic serous cystadenoma and macrocystic (oligocystic) serous cystadenoma, and each has different imaging and gross characteristics.

Imaging Features

Microcystic serous cystadenomas have characteristic findings on imaging studies. By computed tomography (CT) scan, the cysts typically appear as well-defined lesions with a honeycomb pattern of microcysts separated by delicate septa and a centrally located stellate scar with or without a "sunburst" pattern of calcification (**Fig. 1**A).[3,14] Macrocystic serous cystadenomas can mimic pseudocysts or mucinous cysts on CT (**Fig. 2**A); the presence of a lobular cystic lesion with septation supports the diagnosis of a macrocystic serous cystadenoma.[14,15] By magnetic resonance imaging (MRI), serous cysts show low intensity on T1-weighted images and high intensity seen on T2-weighted images, consistent with a cystic structure (see **Fig. 2**B, C).[3] By endoscopic ultrasound (EUS), microcystic serous cystadenomas produce a characteristic "microlacunar" pattern.[14] If cyst fluid analysis is performed, both CEA and amylase levels should be low. Despite the often-typical radiographic appearance of serous cysts in most cases, a definite diagnosis is rendered in as few as 20% of cases.[1,16] Although combined imaging modalities can improve this percentage, fine-needle aspiration identifies diagnostic serous cells in fewer than 20% of cases.[14,16]

Gross Features

Microcystic serous cystadenomas are typically solitary, well-circumscribed lesions that can

Differential Diagnosis
SEROUS CYSTIC NEOPLASMS

- Mucinous cystic neoplasm
- Lymphangioma
- Retention cyst
- Pseudocyst
- Metastatic renal cell carcinoma

Fig. 1. Microcystic serous cystadenoma. (A) On CT, several small microcysts are visible creating a honeycomb appearance (arrows); a central scar is not evident in this example. (B) Grossly, numerous tiny cysts are noted on the cut surface; the main pancreatic duct is uninvolved (bar = 1 cm).

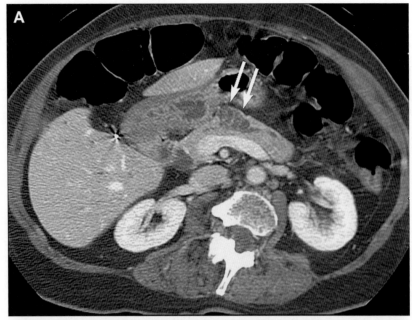

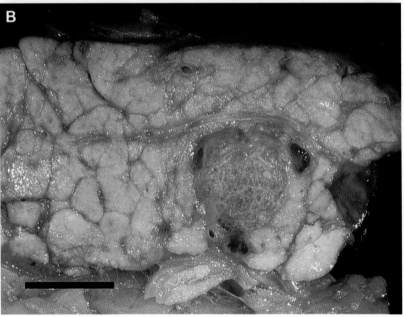

involve any part of the pancreas, but about two-thirds occur in the tail.[2,4] They can range in size from microscopic to larger than 25 cm (mean, 4.9 cm).[4,5] These cysts have a characteristic appearance when sectioned: they are composed of innumerable small, thin-walled cysts with little intervening connective tissue, resembling the cut surface of a sponge or grapefruit (see **Fig. 1**B). The cysts are filled with serous (clear, watery,

pale yellow) fluid. The stellate scar that is often noted radiographically represents centrally located fibrous tissue that may be calcified. Although many of the microcysts are 1 to 3 mm in size, larger cysts can be present near the periphery of the neoplasm. The adjacent pancreatic parenchyma may be normal or atrophic or involved by chronic pancreatitis secondary to mass effect. Although serous

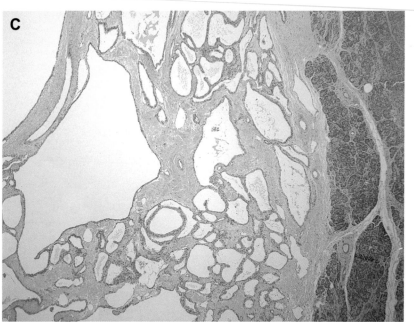

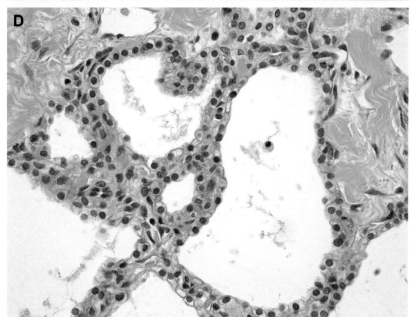

Fig. 1. (*C*) Microscopically, numerous small but variably sized cysts are separated by fibrotic stroma; normal pancreas is present at the right (hematoxylineosin [H&E], original magnification ×40). (*D*) The cysts are lined by bland cuboidal epithelium with clear cytoplasm and centrally located dark, round nuclei (H&E, original magnification ×400).

cystadenomas typically do not communicate with the pancreatic ductal system, cases of ductal communication have been reported.[4,17]

Variations to these typical gross findings can be encountered. Rarely, serous cystadenomas can be composed of one or very few larger (larger than 1 cm) cysts, termed macrocystic or oligocystic serous cystadenoma (see **Fig. 2**E).[18] As mentioned previously, this variant can mimic a mucinous cystic neoplasm or intraductal papillary mucinous neoplasm on imaging studies, making the preoperative diagnosis difficult.[14,15] A similar macrocystic appearance can be caused by cyst degeneration and fibrosis following fine-needle aspiration of a microcystic serous cystadenoma. There is also at least 1 case report of a solid (noncystic) variant.[19]

Fig. 2. Macrocystic serous cyst-adenoma. (*A*) On CT, a 3.7-cm fluid-filled cyst is present within the body of the pancreas (*asterisk*); the CT impression is suspicious for a mucinous cystic neoplasm. (*B*) The cyst shows low intensity on T1-weighted MRI and (*C*) high intensity on T2-weighted MRI images.

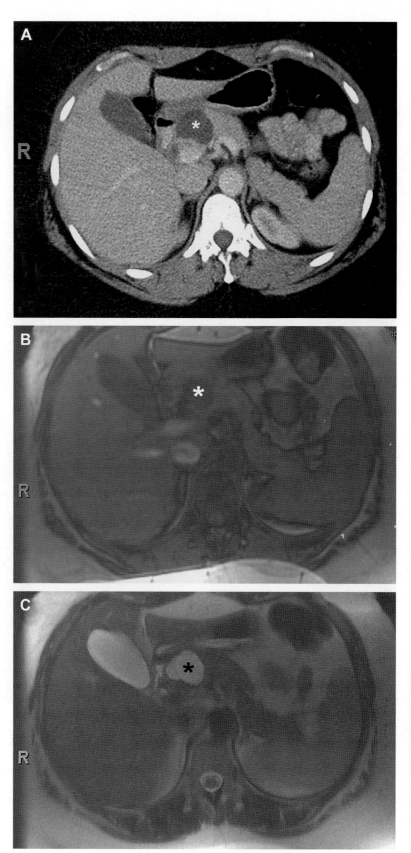

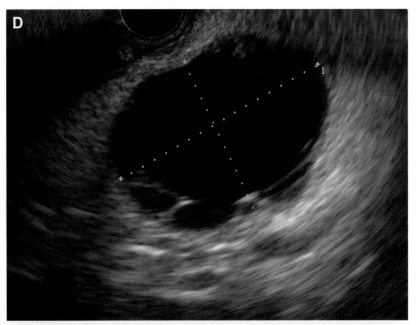

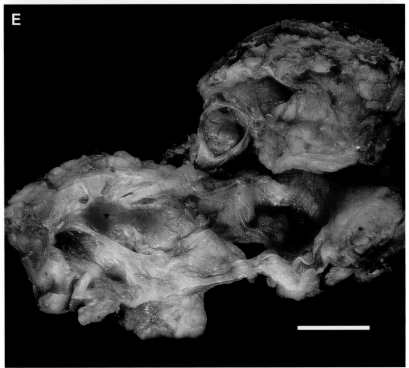

Fig. 2. (*D*) An anechoic cyst with several thinly septated compartments and one main compartment with no internal debris (suspicious for a mucinous cystic neoplasm) is seen on EUS. On MRI and EUS, the contents within the small cysts of a microcystic serous cystadenoma would have features similar to those seen in this macrocystic example. (*E*) Grossly, the large dominant cysts deflate upon sectioning, as occurred in this case. The internal surface is smooth with a single adherent fibrin clot (*asterisk*) (bar = 1 cm).

Microscopic Features

Serous cystadenomas are lined by bland, cuboidal, clear cells with small, centrally located nuclei. Microcystic serous cystadenomas contain numerous small cysts (see **Fig. 1**C, D), whereas the macrocystic variant contains at least 1 large dominant cyst (see **Fig. 2**F, G). The epithelial lining should have minimal to no nuclear atypia, no mitotic activity, and little, if any, cellular pleomorphism. Epithelial tufting and the formation of papillary structures are not typical.

Fig. 2. (*F*) Microscopically, although the cystic spaces are larger than in microcystic serous cystadenomas (H&E, original magnification ×40), (*G*) the epithelial lining is composed of the same bland cuboidal cells with clear cytoplasm and centrally located nuclei (H&E, original magnification ×400).

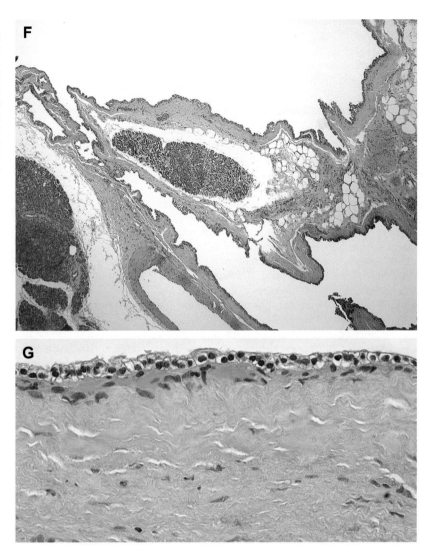

The neoplastic cells are clear because of the presence of intracytoplasmic glycogen, which can be highlighted on a periodic acid–Schiff (PAS) stain (a PAS with diastase stain will be negative, as glycogen is sensitive to diastase). These cells do not contain mucin, so they will be negative for mucin stains, such as mucicarmine, Alcian blue, and the immunohistochemical stains MUC5AC and MUC2. The epithelial cells are immunoreactive for cytokeratins, MUC6, and alpha-inhibin, and occasionally positive (in up to 50% of cases) for MUC1.[20] Importantly, serous cystic lesions should be negative for CEA, both in tissue and cytologic fluid analysis.[1,16,21]

Fibrous stroma of variable thickness separates the individual cysts. This stroma can be pronounced near the center of the cyst, creating the central stellate scar that can become partially calcified. Islets of Langerhans and pancreatic acini can become entrapped within these lesions. Microcystic serous cystadenomas that underwent cystic degeneration following fine-needle aspiration or biopsy may contain evidence of the needle tract (hemosiderin-laden macrophages and/or necrosis) and the larger cystic spaces may be denuded and resemble a pseudocyst at first glance. However, at least a few smaller intact microcysts often remain to aid in the diagnosis of a serous cystic neoplasm.

Prognosis and Treatment

The prognosis for patients with serous cystadenomas of the pancreas is excellent. Although malignant serous cystadenocarcinomas do exist (the definition is based on locally aggressive or metastatic disease, not histopathologic findings), they are exceedingly rare.[22] Complete surgical resection almost always leads to a cure,[3] but smaller, asymptomatic lesions may not require surgical intervention. The main difficulty in determining appropriate treatment is the reliability of the preoperative diagnosis. Unless the diagnosis of a serous cystadenoma is certain, an algorithm for the management of pancreatic cysts of uncertain neoplastic potential should be followed.[23] If a diagnosis of a serous cystadenoma is confirmed, cyst size and presence of symptoms will direct patient care. Resection is recommended for both symptomatic patients and large (larger than 4 cm) serous cystadenomas, regardless if they produce symptoms, whereas patients with incidentally discovered tumors that are smaller than 4 cm in diameter can be observed and followed with periodic imaging.[3,5]

PSEUDOCYST

Background

Pseudocysts are the most common pancreatic cysts,[6] but they are uncommonly encountered in

Key Features
PSEUDOCYST

1. The most common pancreatic cyst

2. An inflammatory (injury-related) cyst that occurs in patients with acute or chronic pancreatitis

3. Cyst fluid amylase and lipase levels are high, whereas CEA is low

4. Typically encountered in surgical pathology when a preoperative diagnosis cannot be confirmed or the patient fails conservative therapy

5. Lacks a true epithelial lining (lined by granulation tissue or fibrous tissue instead)

Differential Diagnosis
PSEUDOCYST

- Mucinous cystic neoplasm
- Macrocystic serous cystadenoma
- Solid pseudopapillary neoplasm
- Solid neoplasm with cystic degeneration
- Parasitic cyst
- Lymphoepithelial cyst

surgical pathology because most are either asymptomatic or can be managed without the need for surgical resection. However, pseudocysts are sometimes resected, typically when the preoperative diagnosis of a benign pseudocyst cannot be confirmed or if the patient fails conservative therapy. Pseudocysts are also sometimes biopsied to exclude a mucinous neoplasm, either as the primary diagnostic procedure, or as sampling of the cyst wall during surgical debridement. Hence, surgical pathologists must be familiar with these non-neoplastic pancreatic cysts.

Pseudocysts are typically encountered in patients with chronic pancreatitis because both pseudocysts and chronic pancreatitis form as the result of prior or recurrent bouts of acute pancreatic injury. Although the highest incidence occurs in chronic pancreatitis owing to alcohol abuse, any cause of acute or chronic pancreatitis, such as gallstone-induced or trauma-related pancreatitis, can result in the formation of pseudocysts.[24] Pseudocysts can also develop in 5% to 16% of patients with acute pancreatitis.[24] During episodes of acute pancreatitis, digestive enzymes are released and autodigest pancreatic and

Pitfalls
PSEUDOCYST

! The wall of a pseudocyst should not contain ducts or other epithelial structures

! If even scant epithelium is present on the surface or in the wall close to the luminal surface, the possibility of a denuded epithelial cyst should be considered

Fig. 3. Pseudocyst. (*A*) On CT, a large fluid-filled cyst with a thick wall is present near the tail of the pancreas (T). (*B*) Grossly, this pseudocyst is located between the tail of the pancreas and the spleen adjacent to the splenic vein (*asterisk*). This cut section demonstrates a thin fibrous wall (pseudocyst walls can be much thicker) with fibrous bands extending into the adjacent fat. Tan-brown necrotic debris is adherent to the internal surface of the cyst. (*C*) Microscopically, the wall of the pseudocyst closest to the lumen (*top*) is composed of fibroblasts, vessels, and scattered lymphocytes; a few macrophages are present on the surface (H&E, original magnification ×100). The wall is more densely fibrotic away from the lumen. Note that there are no normal pancreatic structures within the wall of the pseudocyst (a few atrophic lobules are present deep to the wall of the pseudocyst at the *bottom* of the figure).

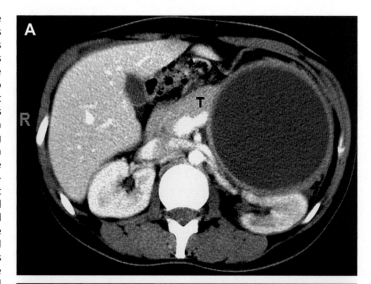

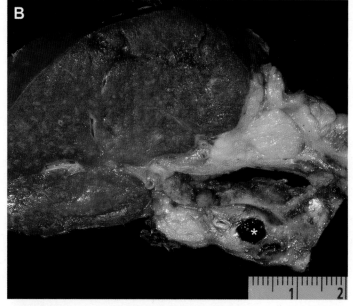

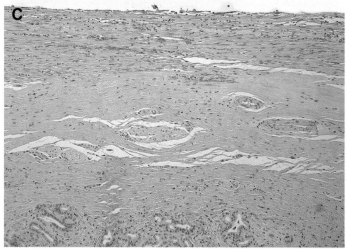

peripancreatic tissue, especially peripancreatic fat. The necrotic tissue is walled-off with the formation of granulation tissue that ultimately becomes densely fibrotic. The necrotic center often liquefies, resulting in a cyst that contains luminal debris and that is devoid of an epithelial lining (hence the name pseudocyst). The cyst fluid has a high concentration of amylase, lipase, and enterokinases, such as trypsin.

Imaging Features

Most pancreatic pseudocysts appear as unilocular fluid-filled cavities. On CT imaging, the cavity is typically surrounded by a dense wall that shows evidence of contrast enhancement (**Fig. 3**A). Nonenhancing zones, representing infection or bleeding, may be present within the cavity. There is often adjacent parenchymal atrophy and/or calcification. The presence of internal dependent debris on MRI is highly specific for pancreatic pseudocysts.[25] By ultrasound, pseudocysts appear as anechoic masses with well-defined borders; infection or hemorrhage can appear as internal echoes or fluid-filled levels.[26]

Gross Features

Pseudocysts are typically found adjacent to the pancreas, but they can involve the pancreatic parenchyma (see **Fig. 3**B). These cysts generally do not communicate with the pancreatic ductal system, but if associated with erosive pancreatitis, a connection with the ductal system can form. They can be of any size and can be multiple. The cyst contents can be watery, viscous, and/or hemorrhagic with or without granular debris; the contents should not appear mucinous. The wall is fibrous and can range from only millimeters to several centimeters in thickness.[18] The internal surface may be smooth and glistening or may appear rough and irregular because of adherent necrotic debris.

Microscopic Features

The microscopic appearance of the pseudocyst wall can vary from predominantly inflammatory (composed of granulation tissue and admixed chronic inflammatory cells and reactive, plump fibroblasts) to densely fibrotic (hyalinized stroma with and scant, spindled fibroblasts) (see **Fig. 3**C). The luminal surface may contain attached necrotic debris and foamy macrophages. Importantly, an epithelial lining is absent. The adjacent pancreas may show evidence of acute or chronic pancreatitis, calcifications, and fat necrosis (saponification).

Some epithelial-lined pancreatic cysts can have densely fibrotic walls and mechanical denudation of the epithelial lining can occur during specimen handling. Hence, if the diagnosis of a pseudocyst has not been confirmed preoperatively, extensive sampling of the wall should be performed to exclude the possibility of an epithelial cyst. The presence of any epithelium within the wall should alert the pathologist that the cyst may be of epithelial origin, because pseudocysts typically do not contain entrapped ductal structures within their walls. Careful inspection of cyst wall biopsies for any evidence of epithelium and/or ovarian-type stroma is required for the same reason.

Prognosis and Treatment

Pseudocysts are benign lesions that resolve spontaneously in 40% to 50% of patients with no serious complications.[27] Hence, if an asymptomatic cyst is determined to be inflammatory in nature, observation is reasonable regardless of size.[23, 27] Intervention is warranted for symptomatic cysts, complicated cysts (such as infected cysts or cysts that compress large vessels or the common bile duct), and progressively growing cysts.[27] Pseudocysts can be drained endoscopically, percutaneously, or surgically (cystgastrostomy or cyst-jejunostomy).[24]

LYMPHOEPITHELIAL CYSTS

Background

Pancreatic lymphoepithelial cysts are benign cysts lined by mature, squamous epithelium with surrounding lymphoid tissue. These cysts tend to occur in middle-aged to older-aged men (male: female ratio 4:1 with a mean age of 56 years).[28] Unlike lymphoepithelial cysts of the head and neck, there are no known associations with conditions such as Sjögren syndrome, human

Key Features
LYMPHOEPITHELIAL CYSTS

1. Benign unilocular or multilocular cyst that resides on or near the surface of the pancreas

2. Often filled with keratinaceous debris

3. Lined by mature squamous epithelium and surrounded by a dense lymphoid stroma; rare sebaceous glands and mucus cells can be present

immunodeficiency virus, or other autoimmune diseases. Most lymphoepithelial cysts are found incidentally on imaging studies and hence the patients are typically asymptomatic, although nonspecific symptoms, such as abdominal pain, nausea, and vomiting, can occur. Although these cysts are nonmucinous and non-neoplastic, cyst fluid CEA and CA19-9 levels can be elevated, a potential pitfall in the preoperative diagnosis of these lesions.[29–31]

Imaging Features

Lymphoepithelial cysts typically appear as multi-locular cysts (and sometimes solid masses) that reside on or near the surface of the pancreas. By CT scan, the cyst contents show decreased atten-uation (**Fig. 4**A).[32] By MRI, the cysts tend to show

high signal intensity on T1-weighted images and granular, low signal intensity on T2-weighted images.[32,33] By EUS, the cysts have internal coarse, heterogeneous hyperechogenicity.[33] These characteristic imaging features likely reflect the lipid and keratin contents of the cysts.

Gross Features

Lymphoepithelial cysts are well-circumscribed cysts that are often multilocular but can be uniloc-ular. They can occur in any part of the pancreas and often protrude outside or appear to reside adjacent to the pancreas (see **Fig. 4**B). The mean size of resected lymphoepithelial cysts is 4.7 cm (range, up to 17.0 cm).[28] The cysts are typically filled with cheesy, tan-white keratinaceous debris that is contained by a thin (1- to 3-mm) fibrous capsule with or without thin septa between varia-bly sized locules.

Microscopic Features

Lymphoepithelial cysts are lined by mature, strati-fied squamous epithelium with areas of keratiniza-tion (see **Fig. 4**C). In nonkeratinizing areas, the squamous epithelium can appear more like "transitional" epithelium with plump superficial squamous cells without keratohyaline granules (see **Fig. 4**C). Rare goblet-shaped mucous cells can be scattered along the epithelial surface (see **Fig. 4**C, inset).[31] Sebaceous glands, but no other adnexal structures, can also be present (see **Fig. 4**D). Immunohistochemically, the squamous epithelium is positive for CK7 and p63, as expected, but the squamous epithelium can also be positive for CEA (see **Fig. 4**E), CA19-9, MUC1, and MUC4, whereas the mucous cells are positive for PAS after diastase, MUC5AC, and MUC4.[31]

The cyst wall and septa just beneath the squa-mous epithelium typically contain abundant lymphoid tissue with lymphoid follicle formation (see **Fig. 4**C). Some lymphoepithelial cysts can be partially or predominantly denuded of the epithelial lining and the wall can sometimes be densely fibrotic with only patchy areas of lymphoid tissue. This finding could be related to prior fine-needle aspiration and can make the diagnosis difficult in the resected specimen. At least focal squamous epithelium and focally dense lymphoid tissue should be present for a definitive diagnosis of a lymphoepithelial cyst.

Prognosis and Treatment

Lymphoepithelial cysts are benign. Although resection is curative, if a definitive diagnosis is

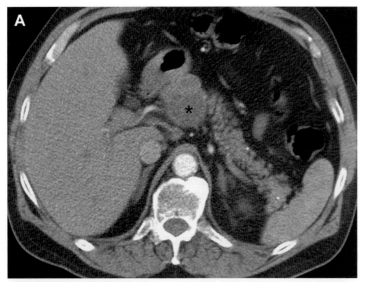

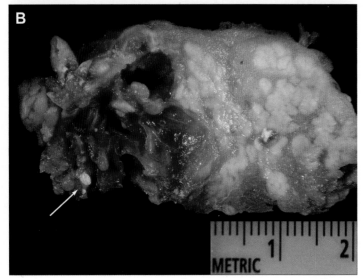

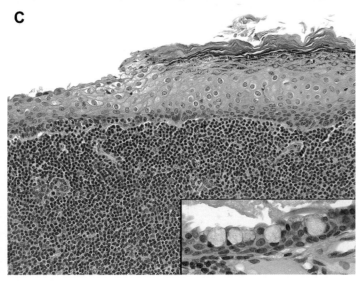

Fig. 4. Lymphoepithelial cyst. (*A*) On CT, a solid-appearing lesion is noted superior to the head of the pancreas (*asterisk*). The lesion is hypovascular and possibly encapsulated with decreased attenuation compared with the capsule. (*B*) Grossly, this lymphoepithelial cyst is multilocular, the cyst wall is tan-brown and the interior surface is smooth. Flecks of yellow, possibly sebaceous material, are present (*arrow*). (*C*) Microscopically, the cyst is lined by stratified squamous epithelium (nonkeratinizing on the left and keratinizing with keratohyaline granules on the right) (H&E, original magnification ×200). Beneath the squamous lining, there is a dense lymphoid infiltrate that can contain germinal centers (not shown). Occasional goblet-shaped mucus cells can be seen within the squamous lining of some lymphoepithelial cysts (inset) (H&E, original magnification ×400).

Fig. 4. (*D*) Sebaceous glands, but no other adnexal structures, can be present (H&E, original magnification ×200). (*E*) The squamous lining is positive for CEA (shown, ×400), CA19-9, MUC1, and MUC4.

D

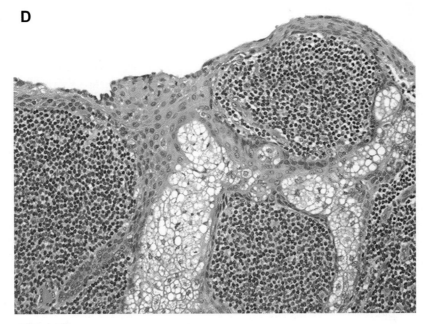

E

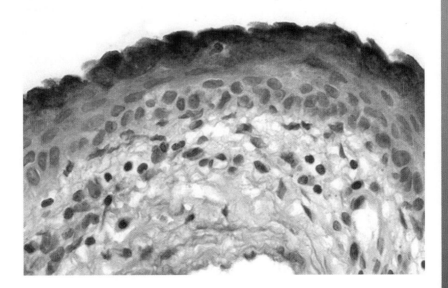

made preoperatively, asymptomatic patients can be observed.[3] If a lymphoepithelial cyst is suspected but the diagnosis is not confirmed or the patient is symptomatic, conservative resection (for easily accessible cysts in the body or tail) is recommended. However, to avoid a pancreaticoduodenectomy for cysts in the head, intraoperative biopsy with internal drainage into a Roux limb of jejunum is a surgical option for these cysts.[3]

RARE/MISCELLANEOUS PANCREATIC CYSTS

Squamoid Cysts

Squamoid cysts of the pancreas were first described by Othman and colleagues[34] in 2007 and in a subsequent case report in 2009.[35] These cysts tend to occur in the head of the pancreas and likely involve and/or arise from the native ductal system. Squamoid cysts can present as discrete lesions on imaging studies

Key Features
RARE/MISCELLANEOUS NONMUCINOUS CYSTS

- *Squamoid cyst:* Squamous-lined cysts that can involve the ductal system

- *Intraductal tubulopapillary neoplasm:* High-grade, nonmucinous, intraductal neoplasm with back-to-back tubules and/or tubulopapillary structures that can obstruct and cystically dilate the pancreatic duct

- *Lymphangioma:* Collection of endothelial-lined cystic spaces with thin septa typically occurring adjacent to the tail of the pancreas

- *Mature cystic teratoma:* Also called a dermoid cyst, they can contain tissues from all 3 germ layers but typically contain sebaceous material and hair

- *Epidermoid cyst in heterotopic spleen:* Squamous-lined cyst surrounded by splenic tissue within the tail of the pancreas

- *Acinar cell cystadenoma:* Pancreatic cysts lined by benign acinar cells

- *True congenital cyst:* Very rare cyst lined by cuboidal epithelium

- *Autosomal dominant polycystic kidney disease:* The pancreas can contain cysts in patients with this disease

- *Cystic fibrosis:* The ducts can become cystically dilated owing to inspissated secretions

- *Parasitic cyst:* Hydatid cysts rarely involve the pancreas

- *Typically solid masses that can present as cystic lesions:* Pancreatic endocrine tumors, solid pseudopapillary neoplasm, ductal adenocarcinoma, acinar cell carcinoma, and metastatic tumors can all have cystic variants

and as incidental findings on pancreatectomy specimens removed for other causes, namely ductal adenocarcinoma.[34] When detected as a specific entity on imaging studies (**Fig. 5**A), these cysts occur at a mean age of 61 years (range, 52 to 80 years). The indications for surgery in these resected cysts include abdominal pain, increasing cyst size, "mass" on imaging studies, and elevated cyst fluid CEA level.

Grossly, squamoid cysts tend to be unilocular with a thin fibrous wall (see **Fig. 5**B). The median size is 1.5 cm (cysts detected preoperatively ranged in size from 0.9 to 9.0 cm with a mean size of 3.2 cm). The cysts can contain clear serous fluid; flecks of off-white material; or hard, white, lumpy material. The adjacent pancreas appears normal. Microscopically, the cysts are lined by variable types of squamoid epithelium including attenuated, flat, squamoid cells; transitional-type epithelium; and stratified squamous epithelium without keratinization (see **Fig. 5**C). Dense, proteinaceous, acellular, eosinophilic material can be present in the lumen. The wall is composed of paucicellular fibrous tissue. Notably absent are mucous, acinar, and endocrine cells; dense lymphoid and ovarian-type stroma within the cyst wall; and surrounding splenic tissue. Immunohistochemically, the squamoid lining is positive for nuclear p63 (in the basal layers), CK7, MUC1, and MUC6. The latter 2 stains support a centroacinar origin. Based on the few cases reported in the literature, squamoid cysts are benign, but as with all cysts in the pancreas, can be challenging to diagnose preoperatively.

Intraductal Tubulopapillary Neoplasm

According to the most recent classification proposed by the World Health Organization, the intraductal neoplasms of the pancreas are separated into 2 groups: (1) intraductal papillary mucinous neoplasms and (2) intraductal tubulopapillary neoplasms (nonmucinous neoplasms that were previously designated as "intraductal tubular neoplasms").[36] Because intraductal tubulopapillary neoplasms arise within dilated pancreatic ducts, these lesions can mimic cystic lesions of the pancreas on preoperative imaging studies and are hence discussed in this article.

Intraductal tubulopapillary neoplasms are rare; they account for fewer than 1% of all pancreatic exocrine neoplasms and only 3% of intraductal neoplasms.[36] These lesions tend to affect men and women equally and the mean age at presentation is about 56 years (range, 35 to 84 years).[36,37] Patients with these lesions may present with vague abdominal complaints or the lesions may be found incidentally. On imaging studies, intraductal tubulopapillary neoplasms typically mimic intraductal papillary mucinous neoplasms. On dynamic CT or MRI, the presence of a hypovascular intraductal mass with lack of delayed enhancement that obstructs the pancreatic duct without downstream pancreatic ductal dilatation may help distinguish these solid intraductal lesions from intraductal papillary mucinous neoplasms.[38] Grossly, intraductal tubulopapillary neoplasms appear as solid nodules that often

Fig. 5. Squamoid cyst. (*A*) This squamoid cyst (*arrow*) forms a discrete cystic structure in the tail of the pancreas that is suspicious for a mucinous cyst. (*B*) Grossly, the cut surface of this cyst appears trabeculated but the lining is smooth and glistening (bar = 1 cm). (*C*) Microscopically, the cyst compresses the adjacent pancreatic parenchyma (H&E, original magnification ×40). Inset: This cyst is lined by stratified nonkeratinizing squamous epithelium that has a transitional appearance (H&E, original magnification ×400).

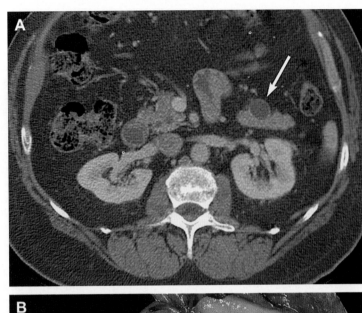

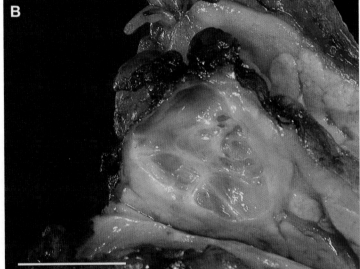

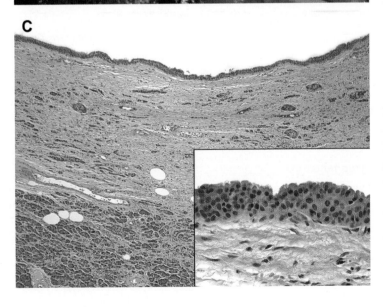

fully occupy and expand the pancreatic duct and show no evidence of mucin production.

Histologically, intraductal tubulopapillary neoplasms are generally uniformly high grade. They are characterized by a tubular growth pattern with complex back-to-back glands and cribriform architecture, papillary and tubulopapillary structures are often present (but may be absent), and solid foci can be seen.[36,37] The neoplastic cells are cuboidal to columnar with eosinophilic-to-amphophilic cytoplasm; the nuclei are enlarged and show moderate to high-grade cytologic atypia. Necrotic foci, including comedo-type necrosis, can be seen, as well as focal stromal desmoplasia within the lesion itself. The lesional cells show evidence of ductal differentiation (as indicated by CK7 and/or CK19 expression), absence of acinar or endocrine differentiation (absence of trypsin and synaptophysin/chromogranin positivity, respectively), and lack overt mucin production (negative staining for MUC2 and MUC5AC). MUC1 and MUC6 are often positive and SMAD4 is typically retained. On a molecular level, mutations in KRAS and BRAF are absent.[37]

The lack of abundant mucin production, prominent cyst formation, and gastric-type or intestinal-type epithelium makes the histologic distinction from most intraductal papillary mucinous neoplasms rather straightforward. The pancreaticobiliary-type of intraductal papillary mucinous neoplasm will lack histologic evidence of mucin production, but these lesions are typically low grade (or have at least areas of low-grade dysplasia) and they typically expressed MUC5AC. One additional entity that is in the differential diagnosis is intraductal tubular adenoma, pyloric gland-type, especially when nonmucinous cuboidal or oncocytic cells are prominent.[39,40] However, these lesions are low grade and should show at least focal or patchy mucin production, as well as MUC5AC positivity.

Prognostic data on intraductal tubulopapillary neoplasms are limited. Even though invasive carcinoma is found in association with about 40% of cases, these appear to be indolent lesions with significantly better prognosis than pancreatic ductal adenocarcinoma.[36,37]

Lymphangioma

Lymphangiomas are rare benign cystic lesions that are thought to represent lymphatic channels that become dilated as the result of congenital or acquired obstruction to lymph flow. Fewer than 1% of lymphangiomas occur in or around the pancreas (most occur in the neck and axillary region).[41] These lesions tend to occur in women at a mean age of 29 years (range, 2 to 61 years).[42] Because pancreatic lymphangiomas can grow quite large (3.0 to 20.0 cm with a mean size of 12.7 cm),[42] patients can present with abdominal pain, nausea and vomiting, or a palpable abdominal mass.

Most lymphangiomas are multicystic and occur in the tail of the pancreas. By CT, lymphangiomas generally appear as well-circumscribed, often encapsulated, water-isodense, polycystic masses with thin septa in or adjacent to the pancreas. They appear as anechoic or hypoechoic, fluid-filled multicystic masses on ultrasound (**Fig. 6**A). Grossly, the cysts have thin walls; a smooth inner lining; and may be filled with clear serous fluid, chylous fluid, or chalky, hemorrhagic fluid. Microscopically, the cystic spaces are lined by flat to slightly raised endothelial cells and may be filled with delicate proteinaceous eosinophilic material (**Fig. 6**B, C). The cystic spaces are surrounded by fibrous tissue that often contains irregular fascicles of smooth muscle, lymphocytes, and foamy histiocytes. The cystic spaces can be present within the pancreatic parenchyma itself or the entire cystic lesion may abut or compress the pancreas. Immunohistochemically, the endothelial cells are positive for CD31, D2-40, and factor VIII-related antigen; CD34 reactivity is variable.[42,43] Pancreatic lymphangiomas are negative for keratin and HMB-45. Similar to other benign pancreatic cysts, a treatment algorithm based on clinicoradiographic features, cyst fluid studies, and certainty of the preoperative diagnosis should be followed. Because many lymphangiomas produce symptoms because of their large size, surgical resection is often performed and the prognosis is excellent.

Mature Cystic Teratoma

The occurrence of mature cystic teratomas (dermoid cysts) in the pancreas is exceedingly rare.[18,44–46] These neoplasms are of germ cell origin and hence generate tissues from all the 3 germ layers (ectoderm, endoderm, and mesoderm). The appearance on imaging studies can be solid or cystic, depending on the types of tissues included in the lesion, but they typically have well-defined borders. Grossly, the cystic nature of the tumor is often evident and the cyst may be filled with sebaceous material and hair. Most reports of mature cystic teratomas in the pancreas describe tumors derived from ectodermal tissue (dermoid cysts) that are lined by squamous epithelium with skin appendages.[18,44–46] The main entity in the differential diagnosis is

Fig. 6. Lymphangioma. (*A*) By EUS, this polycystic lesion adjacent to the tail of the pancreas is anechoic. (*B*) Microscopically, the cystic spaces are separated by delicate septa, some of which contain lymphoid tissue (H&E, original magnification ×40). (*C*) The cystic spaces are lined by flat endothelial cells and the stoma contains lymphocytes and rare smooth muscle fibers (H&E, original magnification ×200).

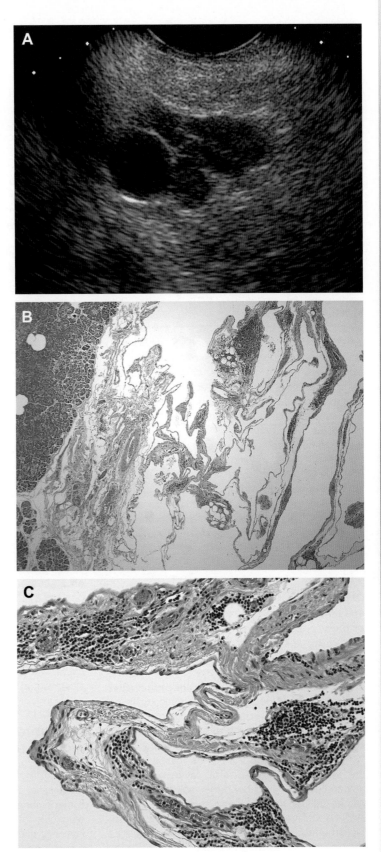

a lymphoepithelial cyst, which can include sebaceous glands but should not include hair or nonsebaceous skin appendages; the characteristic dense lymphoid infiltrate within the wall of lymphoepithelial cysts is lacking in mature cystic teratomas.

Epidermoid Cysts in Heterotopic Spleen

Both splenic epidermoid cysts and intrapancreatic heterotopic spleens are rare, hence the 2 occurring together is extremely rare. However, when they do exist, they can mimic neoplastic mucinous cysts of the pancreas.[47,48] These cysts affect both men and women at a mean age of 47 years (range, 32 to 70 years).[49] Symptoms include abdominal pain, nausea, and weight loss, but about half of the cases in the literature produced no symptoms. All epidermoid cysts in heterotopic spleen have been located in the tail and the mean diameter is 4.8 cm (range, 1.8 to 15.0 cm).[49] On CT, these cysts appear round with well-defined borders and are of higher density than the adjacent pancreas and of the same density as the spleen, features that can mimic a pancreatic endocrine neoplasm.[48] Recent studies show that superparamagnetic iron oxide–enhanced MRI can detect the splenic tissue surrounding the epidermoid cyst in the pancreas.[48] These cysts contain serous fluid or keratinaceous debris and are lined by stratified squamous epithelium that can be keratinizing or nonkeratinizing and can resemble transitional epithelium.[49] The defining feature is the presence of splenic tissue that surrounds the cystic structures.

Acinar Cell Cystadenoma

The term acinar cell cystadenoma applies to one or more cysts in the pancreas that are lined by benign acinar cells.[50–52] The mean age at diagnosis is 47 years, but at least one cyst has been reported in a child.[53] These cysts, which can be found incidentally or can cause abdominal pain, can mimic other neoplastic pancreatic cysts on imaging studies. Grossly, the cysts can be unilocular or multilocular and can range up to 15 cm in diameter; rarely, they can involve the entire pancreas.[50] Microscopically, the cystic spaces are lined by one to several layers of benign acinar cells. Similar to normal acinar cells, the acinar cells lining the cystic spaces will contain PAS-D–positive granules and will react immunohistochemically to acinar cell markers, such as trypsin, chymotrypsin, and lipase.

True Congenital Cysts

True single congenital cysts of the pancreas are very rare and are most often seen in infant girls.[54] They are located in the body and tail of the pancreas and can range up to 5 cm in diameter. These cysts can resemble retention cysts, as they are typically lined by cuboidal (ductal-type) epithelium; however, these cysts generally do not communicate with the pancreatic duct. Although the multiple cysts of VHL disease are often described as congenital in nature, their glycogen-rich clear cell lining suggests these may represent serous cystadenomas rather than true congenital cysts.[18]

Autosomal Dominant Polycystic Kidney Disease

Although renal cysts are the characteristic feature of this disease, cysts may be found in the liver, spleen, adrenal glands, and pancreas. Pancreatic cysts are present in about 9% of patients older than 30.[55]

Cystic Fibrosis

Pancreatic ducts in patients with cystic fibrosis can become dilated and cystlike owing to inspissated secretions and the ensuing inflammatory response. Typically, there are variable numbers of cysts that range from 1 to 3 mm in size and generally do not exceed 5 cm in diameter. In rare instances, the entire pancreas can become replaced by multiple macroscopic cysts, termed "pancreatic cystosis."[56]

Parasitic Cyst

Hydatid cysts rarely occur in the pancreas.[57–59] When present, a hydatid cyst typically presents as a single, unilocular or multilocular cyst in the head of the gland, which can mimic a mucinous cyst or a pseudocyst.[57,58] This entity should be included in the differential diagnosis if the patient has traveled to an area where echinococcal disease is endemic. Although pancreatic hydatid cysts can be treated medically, surgery is the treatment of choice.

TYPICALLY SOLID MASSES THAT CAN PRESENT AS CYSTIC LESIONS OR CONTAIN A CYSTIC COMPONENT

Pancreatic Endocrine Neoplasm

Pancreatic endocrine neoplasms can present as cystic lesions and must be included in the differential diagnosis of pancreatic cysts. Because several layers of endocrine cells typically line these cysts, a cystic pancreatic endocrine neoplasm can often

Fig. 7. Cystic pancreatic endocrine neoplasm. (*A*) On CT, this fluid-filled cyst in the pancreatic tail (*arrow*) has a thick, partially enhancing outer wall. (*B*) Grossly, the cyst has a thick, tan-brown lining that is surrounded by a fibrous wall. The interior surface is smooth and has increased vascularity. (*C*) Microscopically, several layers of neoplastic endocrine cells (*top left*) line the cyst (H&E, original magnification ×100). A dense fibrous wall separates the cyst lining from the adjacent pancreas (*lower right*).

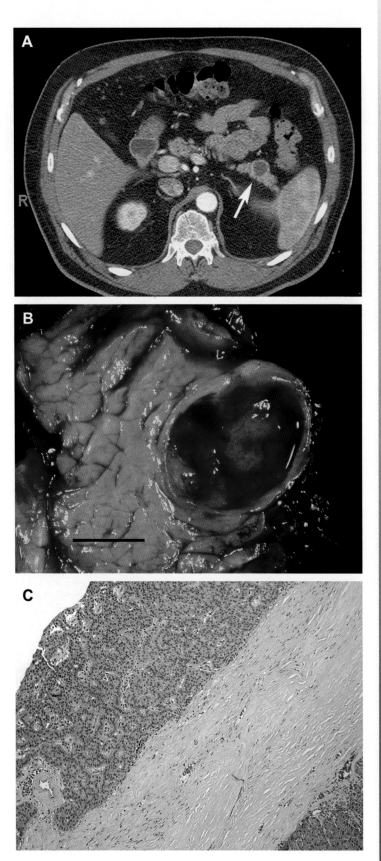

be diagnosed on imaging studies as a fluid-filled cyst with a thick, sometimes hypervascular wall (**Fig. 7**A). Resected cystic pancreatic endocrine neoplasms are typically well circumscribed and contain watery or hemorrhagic fluid surrounded by a rim of tan-brown tissue (see **Fig. 7**B). Microscopically, these tumors are indistinguishable from their solid counterparts (see **Fig. 7**C), but occasionally the neoplastic endocrine cells are scarce and multiple sections may be needed to make this diagnosis. Both primary pancreatic malignancies, including ductal adenocarcinomas and acinar cell carcinomas, and metastatic malignancies, including renal cell carcinoma and ovarian carcinoma, can produce cystic lesions.[2]

Solid Pseudopapillary Neoplasm

Solid pseudopapillary neoplasms are covered in the article by Ohike and Toshio elsewhere in this issue. It is important to note here that these non-mucinous tumors often contain cystic areas owing to cellular degeneration and necrosis and can present as cystic pancreatic lesions or masses.

DUODENAL CYSTS THAT CAN INVOLVE/ABUT THE PANCREAS

Paraduodenal Pancreatitis with Cyst Formation

Paraduodenal pancreatitis is a form of chronic pancreatitis that involves pancreatic tissue in and around the duodenal wall, particularly near the minor papilla.[60–62] Because paraduodenal

Key Features
DUODENAL CYSTS THAT CAN INVOLVE/ABUT THE PANCREAS

- *Paraduodenal pancreatitis with cyst formation:* A form of pancreatitis that typically creates cysts lined by cuboidal or columnar epithelium (or denuded of epithelium) within or adjacent to a thickened duodenal wall

- *Duodenal diverticulum:* Typically occurs in the periampullary region and can mimic a pancreatic cyst on imaging studies

- *Duplication cyst:* Also called a foregut cyst or enteric cyst, can be lined by small intestinal, gastric, squamous, or ciliated columnar epithelium with surrounding smooth muscle; can abut or compress the pancreas

pancreatitis is covered in the article by Farris III and colleagues elsewhere in this issue, it will be only briefly mentioned here in the context of cyst formation. The cysts that form are thought to represent dilated ducts that become denuded and inflamed, resulting in cystic structures that can resemble pseudocysts. Grossly, cystic structures that can range up to 2 cm in diameter are noted within or adjacent to a thickened duodenal wall (**Fig. 8**A). The cysts can contain clear fluid, granular white material, and stones. Microscopically, cysts, often with inspissated eosinophilic secretions, are present within the duodenal submucosa and muscular wall (see **Fig. 8**B). Pancreatic acini and islets may or may not be present (if present, they are thought to represent pancreatic heterotopia). The larger cysts are often devoid of an epithelial lining (see **Fig. 8**B), but the smaller cysts can be lined by ductal (cuboidal or mucinous) epithelium (see **Fig. 8**C). The wall of the cysts can be composed of organizing granulation tissue with a marked inflammatory response or dense fibrosis.

Duodenal Diverticula

Duodenal diverticula typically occur in the periampullary region and most patients are asymptomatic. Similar to colonic diverticula, most duodenal diverticula are acquired rather than congenital. Occasionally, duodenal diverticula can mimic cystic neoplasms of the pancreas.[63,64] On imaging studies, when a cystic process is noted to reside adjacent to the pancreatic head and the second portion of the duodenum, a duodenal diverticulum should be in the differential diagnosis (**Fig. 9**A). Small amounts of gas or air-fluid levels, especially on MRI, support this diagnosis.[63] A barium swallow examination can help confirm the diagnosis. If resected, duodenal diverticula appear similar to diverticula elsewhere in the gastrointestinal tract and should be lined by duodenal mucosa that is in continuity with duodenal lumen (see **Fig. 9**B, C).

Duplication Cysts (Foregut Cyst)

Duplication cysts (also called enteric cysts or foregut cysts) are benign congenital cysts that often present in childhood and can cause pancreatitis when they arise from the duodenum or stomach.[2,18,65] As opposed to diverticula, duplication cysts typically arise within the wall of the duodenum (or stomach) and can compress the pancreas.[66] They typically do not communicate with the luminal gastrointestinal tract or the pancreatic duct. Duplication cysts can be lined by

Fig. 8. Paraduodenal pancreatitis with cyst formation. (*A*) Grossly, a cystic space with a smooth internal surface surrounded by dense fibrosis resides in the "groove" between the pancreas (*top*) and the duodenum (*asterisk* = duodenal lumen). (*B*) Microscopically, a large cystic space is present within a thickened duodenal wall (Brunner glands are present in the *upper right*). The cystic space is predominantly denuded and contains an inflammatory exudate on the surface; one cluster of detached epithelial cells are present (*upper left*) (H&E, original magnification ×40). (*C*) Smaller cysts within the duodenal wall are lined by reactive cuboidal-to-columnar epithelial cells and inflammatory cells are present in the lumen; another cystic space devoid of an epithelial lining is present in the lower right corner (H&E, original magnification ×100).

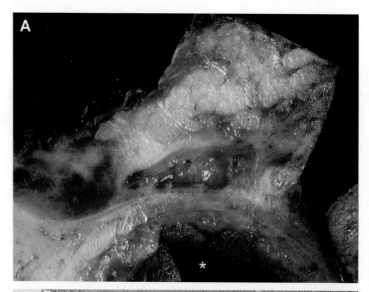

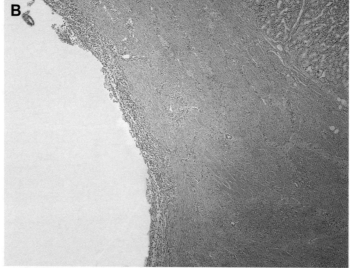

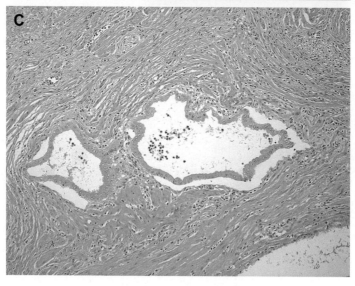

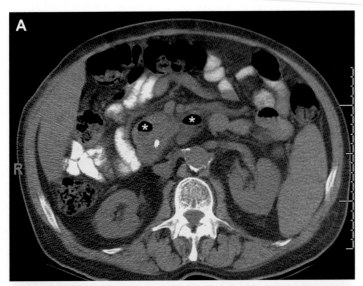

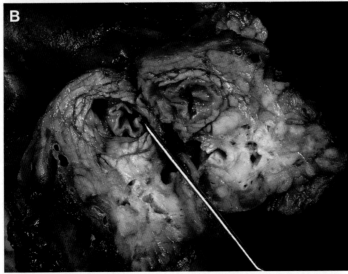

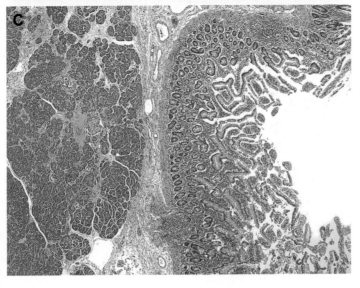

Fig. 9. Duodenal diverticulum. (*A*) On CT, this patient has 2 duodenal diverticula (*asterisk*) that create air-filled cystic spaces that appear to reside within the pancreas. If these diverticula were filled with fluid, they could mimic pancreatic cysts. (*B*) Grossly, this bisected Whipple specimen demonstrates a duodenal diverticulum that is surrounded by pancreatic parenchyma but is lined by tan, regularly folded duodenal mucosa (the metal probe proceeds into the duodenal lumen). (*C*) Microscopically, normal duodenal mucosa and muscularis mucosae (*right*) have protruded beyond the duodenal muscularis propria and lie adjacent to normal pancreas (*left*) (H&E, original magnification ×40).

Fig. 10. This duodenal duplication cyst has an irregular muscle wall with a lining composed of ciliated columnar epithelium with rare goblet cells (inset) (H&E, original magnification ×100; inset, ×400).

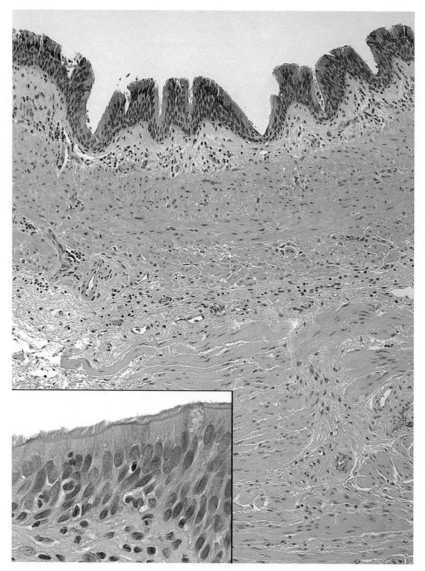

small intestinal, gastric, squamous, and/or ciliated columnar epithelium and contain organized fascicles of smooth muscle in the wall (**Fig. 10**).[2,18]

REFERENCES

1. Vignesh S, Brugge WR. Endoscopic diagnosis and treatment of pancreatic cysts. J Clin Gastroenterol 2008;42(5):493–506.

2. Basturk O, Coban I, Adsay NV. Pancreatic cysts: pathologic classification, differential diagnosis, and clinical implications. Arch Pathol Lab Med 2009; 133(3):423–38.

3. Katz MH, Mortenson MM, Wang H, et al. Diagnosis and management of cystic neoplasms of the pancreas: an evidence-based approach. J Am Coll Surg 2008;207(1):106–20.

4. Le Borgne J, de Calan L, Partensky C. Cystadenomas and cystadenocarcinomas of the pancreas: a multiinstitutional retrospective study of 398 cases. French Surgical Association. Ann Surg 1999;230(2): 152–61.

5. Tseng JF, Warshaw AL, Sahani DV, et al. Serous cystadenoma of the pancreas: tumor growth rates and recommendations for treatment. Ann Surg 2005; 242(3):413–9 [discussion: 419–21].

6. Kosmahl M, Pauser U, Peters K, et al. Cystic neoplasms of the pancreas and tumor-like lesions with cystic features: a review of 418 cases and a classification proposal. Virchows Arch 2004;445(2):168–78.

7. Solcia E, Capella C, Kloppel G. Tumors of the pancreas. Atlas of tumor pathology, 3rd Series, Fascicle 20. Washington, DC: Armed Forces Institute of Pathology; 1997.

8. Wargo JA, Fernandez-del-Castillo C, Warshaw AL. Management of pancreatic serous cystadenomas. Adv Surg 2009;43:23–34.

9. Horton WA, Wong V, Eldridge R. Von Hippel-Lindau disease: clinical and pathological manifestations in nine families with 50 affected members. Arch Intern Med 1976;136(7):769–77.

10. Levine E, Collins DL, Horton WA, et al. CT screening of the abdomen in von Hippel-Lindau disease. AJR Am J Roentgenol 1982;139(3):505–10.

11. Mukhopadhyay B, Sahdev A, Monson JP, et al. Pancreatic lesions in von Hippel-Lindau disease. Clin Endocrinol (Oxf) 2002;57(5):603–8.

12. Hough DM, Stephens DH, Johnson CD, et al. Pancreatic lesions in von Hippel-Lindau disease: prevalence, clinical significance, and CT findings. AJR Am J Roentgenol 1994;162(5):1091–4.

13. Lonser RR, Glenn GM, Walther M, et al. von Hippel-Lindau disease. Lancet 2003;361(9374):2059–67.

14. Procacci C, Graziani R, Bicego E, et al. Serous cystadenoma of the pancreas: report of 30 cases with emphasis on the imaging findings. J Comput Assist Tomogr 1997;21(3):373–82.

15. Kim SY, Lee JM, Kim SH, et al. Macrocystic neoplasms of the pancreas: CT differentiation of serous oligocystic adenoma from mucinous cystadenoma and intraductal papillary mucinous tumor. AJR Am J Roentgenol 2006;187(5):1192–8.

16. Belsley NA, Pitman MB, Lauwers GY, et al. Serous cystadenoma of the pancreas: limitations and pitfalls of endoscopic ultrasound-guided fine-needle aspiration biopsy. Cancer 2008;114(2):102–10.

17. Samel S, Horst F, Becker H, et al. Serous adenoma of the pancreas with multiple microcysts communicating with the pancreatic duct. HPB Surg 1998; 11(1):43–9.

18. Hruban RH, Pitman MB, Klimstra DS. Tumors of the pancreas. Atlas of tumor pathology, 4th Series, Fascicle 6. Washington, DC: Armed Forces Institute of Pathology; 2007.

19. Perez-Ordonez B, Naseem A, Lieberman PH, et al. Solid serous adenoma of the pancreas. The solid variant of serous cystadenoma? Am J Surg Pathol 1996;20(11):1401–5.

20. Kosmahl M, Wagner J, Peters K, et al. Serous cystic neoplasms of the pancreas: an immunohistochemical analysis revealing alpha-inhibin, neuron-specific enolase, and MUC6 as new markers. Am J Surg Pathol 2004;28(3):339–46.

21. Ishikawa T, Nakao A, Nomoto S, et al. Immunohistochemical and molecular biological studies of serous cystadenoma of the pancreas. Pancreas 1998; 16(1):40–4.

22. King JC, Ng TT, White SC, et al. Pancreatic serous cystadenocarcinoma: a case report and review of the literature. J Gastrointest Surg 2009;13(10):1864–8.

23. Turner BG, Brugge WR. Pancreatic cystic lesions: when to watch, when to operate, and when to ignore. Curr Gastroenterol Rep 2010;12(2):98–105.

24. Aghdassi A, Mayerle J, Kraft M, et al. Diagnosis and treatment of pancreatic pseudocysts in chronic pancreatitis. Pancreas 2008;36(2):105–12.

25. Macari M, Finn ME, Bennett GL, et al. Differentiating pancreatic cystic neoplasms from pancreatic pseudocysts at MR imaging: value of perceived internal debris. Radiology 2009;251(1):77–84.

26. Ros PR, Hamrick-Turner JE, Chiechi MV, et al. Cystic masses of the pancreas. Radiographics 1992;12(4): 673–86.

27. Gumaste VV, Aron J. Pseudocyst management: endoscopic drainage and other emerging techniques. J Clin Gastroenterol 2010;44(5):326–31.

28. Adsay NV, Hasteh F, Cheng JD, et al. Lymphoepithelial cysts of the pancreas: a report of 12 cases and a review of the literature. Mod Pathol 2002;15(5): 492–501.

29. Centeno BA, Stockwell JW, Lewandrowski KB. Cyst fluid cytology and chemical features in a case of lymphoepithelial cyst of the pancreas: a rare and difficult preoperative diagnosis. Diagn Cytopathol 1999;21(5):328–30.

30. Yamaguchi T, Takahashi H, Kagawa R, et al. Lymphoepithelial cyst of the pancreas associated with elevated CA 19-9 levels. J Hepatobiliary Pancreat Surg 2008;15(6):652–4.

31. Raval JS, Zeh HJ, Moser AJ, et al. Pancreatic lymphoepithelial cysts express CEA and can contain mucous cells: potential pitfalls in the preoperative diagnosis. Mod Pathol 2010;23(11):1467–76.

32. Fukukura Y, Inoue H, Miyazono N, et al. Lymphoepithelial cysts of the pancreas: demonstration of lipid component using CT and MRI. J Comput Assist Tomogr 1998;22(2):311–3.

33. Shinmura R, Gabata T, Matsui O. Lymphoepithelial cyst of the pancreas: case report with special reference to imaging–pathologic correlation. Abdom Imaging 2006;31(1):106–9.

34. Othman M, Basturk O, Groisman G, et al. Squamoid cyst of pancreatic ducts: a distinct type of cystic lesion in the pancreas. Am J Surg Pathol 2007; 31(2):291–7.

35. Kurahara H, Shinchi H, Mataki Y, et al. A case of squamoid cyst of pancreatic ducts. Pancreas 2009;38(3):349–51.

36. Adsay NV, Fukushima N, Furukawa T, et al. Intraductal neoplasms of the pancreas. In: Bosman FT, Carneiro F, Hruban RH, et al, editors. WHO classification of tumours of the digestive system. 4th edition. Lyon (France): IARC Press; 2010. p. 304–14.

37. Yamaguchi H, Shimizu M, Ban S, et al. Intraductal tubulopapillary neoplasms of the pancreas distinct from pancreatic intraepithelial neoplasia and intraductal papillary mucinous neoplasms. Am J Surg Pathol 2009;33(8):1164–72.

38. Ishigami K, Yoshimitsu K, Irie H, et al. Imaging of intraductal tubular tumors of the pancreas. AJR Am J Roentgenol 2008;191(6):1836–40.

39. Albores-Saavedra J, Sheahan K, O'Riain C, et al. Intraductal tubular adenoma, pyloric type, of the pancreas: additional observations on a new type of pancreatic neoplasm. Am J Surg Pathol 2004;28(2):233–8.

40. Chetty R, Serra S. Intraductal tubular adenoma (pyloric gland-type) of the pancreas: a reappraisal and possible relationship with gastric-type intraductal papillary mucinous neoplasm. Histopathology 2009;55(3):270–6.

41. Leung TK, Lee CM, Shen LK, et al. Differential diagnosis of cystic lymphangioma of the pancreas based on imaging features. J Formos Med Assoc 2006;105(6):512–7.

42. Paal E, Thompson LD, Heffess CS. A clinicopathologic and immunohistochemical study of ten pancreatic lymphangiomas and a review of the literature. Cancer 1998;82(11):2150–8.

43. Hornick JL, Fletcher CD. Intraabdominal cystic lymphangiomas obscured by marked superimposed reactive changes: clinicopathological analysis of a series. Hum Pathol 2005;36(4):426–32.

44. Koomalsingh KJ, Fazylov R, Chorost MI, et al. Cystic teratoma of the pancreas: presentation, evaluation and management. JOP 2006;7(6):643–6.

45. Seki M, Ninomiya E, Aruga A, et al. Image-diagnostic features of mature cystic teratomas of the pancreas: report on two cases difficult to diagnose preoperatively. J Hepatobiliary Pancreat Surg 2005;12(4):336–40.

46. Tucci G, Muzi MG, Nigro C, et al. Dermoid cyst of the pancreas: presentation and management. World J Surg Oncol 2007;5:85.

47. Gleeson FC, Kendrick ML, Chari ST, et al. Epidermoid accessory splenic cyst masquerading as a pancreatic mucinous cystic neoplasm. Endoscopy 2008;40(Suppl 2):E141–2.

48. Motosugi U, Yamaguchi H, Ichikawa T, et al. Epidermoid cyst in intrapancreatic accessory spleen: radiological findings including superparamagnetic iron oxide-enhanced magnetic resonance imaging. J Comput Assist Tomogr 2010;34(2):217–22.

49. Kadota K, Kushida Y, Miyai Y, et al. Epidermoid cyst in an intrapancreatic accessory spleen: three case reports and review of the literatures. Pathol Oncol Res 2010;16(3):435–42.

50. Zamboni G, Terris B, Scarpa A, et al. Acinar cell cystadenoma of the pancreas: a new entity? Am J Surg Pathol 2002;26(6):698–704.

51. Kloppel G. Pseudocysts and other non-neoplastic cysts of the pancreas. Semin Diagn Pathol 2000; 17(1):7–15.

52. Albores-Saavedra J. Acinar cystadenoma of the pancreas: a previously undescribed tumor. Ann Diagn Pathol 2002;6(2):113–5.

53. McEvoy MP, Rich B, Klimstra D, et al. Acinar cell cystadenoma of the pancreas in a 9-year-old boy. J Pediatr Surg 2010;45(5):e7–9.

54. Auringer ST, Ulmer JL, Sumner TE, et al. Congenital cyst of the pancreas. J Pediatr Surg 1993;28(12): 1570–1.

55. Torra R, Nicolau C, Badenas C, et al. Ultrasonographic study of pancreatic cysts in autosomal dominant polycystic kidney disease. Clin Nephrol 1997;47(1):19–22.

56. Hernanz-Schulman M, Teele RL, Perez-Atayde A, et al. Pancreatic cystosis in cystic fibrosis. Radiology 1986;158(3):629–31.

57. Yorganci K, Iret D, Sayek I. A case of primary hydatid disease of the pancreas simulating cystic neoplasm. Pancreas 2000;21(1):104–5.

58. Bayat AM, Azhough R, Hashemzadeh S, et al. Hydatid cyst of pancreas presented as a pancreatic pseudocyst. Am J Gastroenterol 2009;104(5):1324–6.

59. Khiari A, Mzali R, Ouali M, et al. Hydatid cyst of the pancreas. Apropos of 7 cases. Ann Gastroenterol Hepatol (Paris) 1994;30(3):87–91 [in French].

60. Adsay NV, Zamboni G. Paraduodenal pancreatitis: a clinico-pathologically distinct entity unifying "cystic dystrophy of heterotopic pancreas," "paraduodenal wall cyst," and "groove pancreatitis". Semin Diagn Pathol 2004;21(4):247–54.

61. Tezuka K, Makino T, Hirai I, et al. Groove pancreatitis. Dig Surg 2010;27(2):149–52.

62. Zamboni G, Capelli P, Scarpa A, et al. Nonneoplastic mimickers of pancreatic neoplasms. Arch Pathol Lab Med 2009;133(3):439–53.

63. Macari M, Lazarus D, Israel G, et al. Duodenal diverticula mimicking cystic neoplasms of the pancreas: CT and MR imaging findings in seven patients. AJR Am J Roentgenol 2003;180(1):195–9.

64. Mazziotti S, Costa C, Ascenti G, et al. MR cholangiopancreatography diagnosis of juxtapapillary duodenal diverticulum simulating a cystic lesion of the pancreas: usefulness of an oral negative contrast agent. AJR Am J Roentgenol 2005;185(2): 432–5.

65. Guarise A, Faccioli N, Ferrari M, et al. Duodenal duplication cyst causing severe pancreatitis: imaging findings and pathological correlation. World J Gastroenterol 2006;12(10):1630–3.

66. Nijs E, Callahan MJ, Taylor GA. Disorders of the pediatric pancreas: imaging features. Pediatr Radiol 2005;35(4):358–73 [quiz: 457].

Key Features
HISTOLOGIC FEATURES OF NONDUCTAL NEOPLASMS

Acinar cell carcinoma

- Marked cellularity
- Acinar differentiation
  - Acinar units
  - Basal nuclear polarization
  - Chromophilic and granular cytoplasm
  - Large, central, single nucleoli

Pancreatoblastoma

- Multiple lines of differentiation
- Squamoid nests

Solid-pseudopapillary neoplasm

- Poor cohesiveness
- Pseudopapillae
- Foam cells
- Hyaline globules
- Nuclear grooves

Helpful Markers of Immunohistochemistry for Nonductal Neoplasms

Acinar cell carcinoma

- Trypsin, chymotrypsin, cytokeratins (8 and 18)

Pancreatoblastoma

- Acinar markers (trypsin, chymotrypsin, and so forth)
- Endocrine markers (chromogranin, synaptophysin)
- Ductal markers (CEA, B72.3, and so forth) in the corresponding components
- Abnormal (nuclear and cytoplasmic) β-catenin expression in squamoid nests

Solid-pseudopapillary neoplasm

- Vimentin, α-1-antitryipsin (not to be confused with trypsin), CD10, CD56, progesterone receptor, abnormal (nuclear and cytoplasmic) β-catenin expression

resemblance to pancreatic acinar cells. Most patients are adults (mean, 58 years), but some occur in children. ACCs represent 1% to 2% of exocrine pancreatic neoplasms in adults and 15% in children. Males are affected more frequently and no preferential localization is seen.[1,2] Presenting symptoms are usually nonspecific and related to local tumor growth or metastases. The most common complaint is abdominal pain. Rare paraneoplastic syndrome called *lipase hypersecretion syndrome* occurs mainly in patients with hepatic metastases.[1,2] Serum alpha-fetoprotein (AFP) levels may be elevated.

GROSS FEATURES

ACC most often present as a large, well-demarcated, soft, round to sausagelike mass that might be partially or completely encapsulated.[3] Its size ranges from 2 to 30 cm with a mean of 10 cm.[1] The cut surface is tan to reddish, and fleshy. Thin, fibrous strands separating the tumor into large lobules might be seen grossly (**Fig. 1A**). Necrosis and degenerative cystic changes are often present (see **Fig. 1B**), which lead to a heterogeneous appearance on radiological images. Some extend into the pancreatic duct, forming polypoid nodules, which may be detected as filling defects of the pancreatic duct on endoscopic retrograde pancreatography. Tumors often infiltrate into adjacent structures, such as duodenum, spleen, stomach, or major vessels.

MICROSCOPIC FEATURES

ACCs are usually well-circumscribed neoplasms composed of highly cellular nodules separated by hypocellular fibrous bands. Necrosis might be present. Of the described histologic growth patterns, the most common are acinar and solid patterns, and these are usually seen together. Acinar pattern is characterized by small acinar units that have small lumens surrounded by basally located nuclei (**Fig. 2A**). In some instances, the lumens are more dilated, resulting in a glandular pattern or cystic formation. A solid pattern represents proliferation of neoplastic cells in sheets and nests (**Fig. 3A**). Therefore, fine-needle aspiration usually reveals a high cellular yield containing numerous individual neoplastic cells and cells arranged in small glandular clusters or irregular solid sheets.[2] The tumor cells are characterized by moderate to abundant amounts of chromophilic (basophilic to eosinophilic) cytoplasm and uniform round to oval nuclei with single prominent nucleoli (see **Figs. 2A and 3A**). Apical cytoplasmic granularity (diastase-resistant periodic acid Schiff [PAS]-positive), reflecting the presence of zymogen granules, is detectable, but may be minimal. The mitotic rate is variable by cases, but is usually more than 10 per 10 high power fields. Vascular and perineural invasion

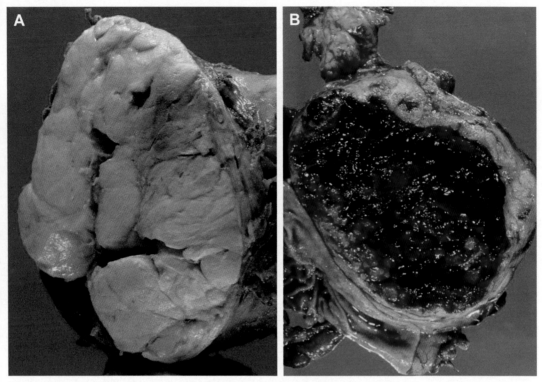

Fig. 1. Acinar cell carcinoma. The tumor is forming an encapsulated expansile mass showing a gray, lobulated solid cut surface (*A*). Cystic change owing to hemorrhagic necrosis is often seen (*B*).

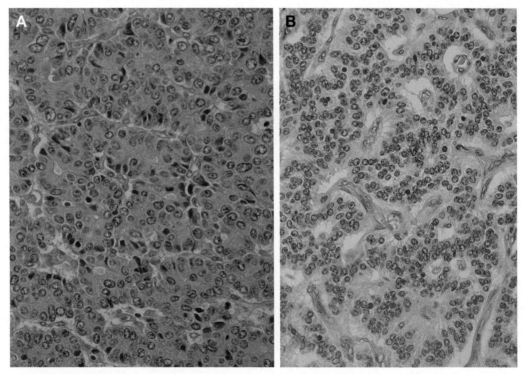

Fig. 2. Pancreatic acinar cell carcinoma (*A*) and neuroendocrine tumor (*B*) showing acinar/trabecular growth. In acinar cell carcinoma, basal nuclear polarization of tumor cells is more prominent and the cytoplasm is more chromophilic (hematoxylin and eosin [H&E] stain, original magnification ×400).

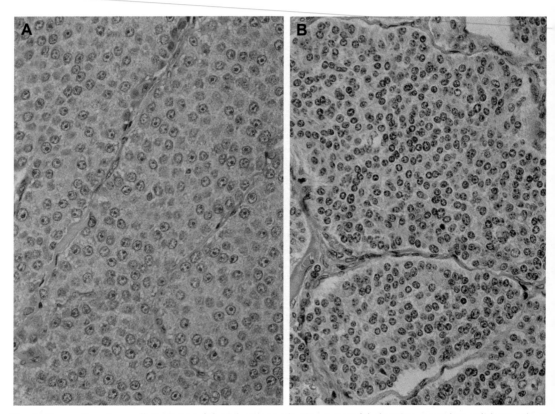

Fig. 3. Pancreatic acinar cell carcinoma (*A*) and neuroendocrine tumor (*B*) showing nested to solid growth. In acinar cell carcinoma, tumor cells show more prominent single, central nucleoli and the cytoplasm looks more granular (H&E stain, original magnification ×400).

are common. Ultrastructurally, most neoplastic cells contain electron-dense, round zymogen granules (ranging from 125 to 1000 nm) and irregular fibrillary granules. Immunohistochemically, ACCs are almost always positive for CAM 5.2 and AE1/AE3 (owing to CK8 and CK18 production) and express several markers of acinar differentiation, including trypsin, chymotrypsin, lipase, and phospholipase.[1,2,4] Among these, trypsin is currently the most frequently used and reliable marker.[1,2] The immunolabeling may be patchy. Some cases may also show focal (by definition <25% of the tumor cells) positivity with endocrine markers.[5]

VARIANTS

Acinar cell cystadenocarcinomas are rare, grossly cystic neoplasms with innumerable variably sized cysts, lined by layers of atypical neoplastic cells with acinar differentiation.[1,2] Most cases present with a large tumor (mean, 24 cm).

Intraductal and papillary variant is a recently described subtype of ACC with intraductal papillary growth and cystic dilation of ducts.[6] They

mimic intraductal papillary-mucinous neoplasms or intraductal tubulo-papillary neoplasms.

Mixed acinar carcinomas are considered as ACCs with a substantial proportion (>25% of the tumor) of neuroendocrine and/or ductal component and are called, depending on the cell types identified, "mixed acinar-neuroendocrine carcinoma" (probably the most common mixed carcinoma subtype), "mixed acinar-ductal carcinoma," or "mixed acinar-neuroendocrine-ductal carcinoma."[2,5,7] Neuroendocrine or ductal differentiation is recognized by a thorough histologic and immunohistochemical evaluation. By definition, metastases also follow the same mixed features.

DIFFERENTIAL DIAGNOSIS

Pancreatic neoplasms with extensive acinar differentiation include ACC and PB. These neoplasms have histologic similarity and, in addition, share several genetic events. Thus, PB is regarded as the pediatric form of ACC. Squamoid nest is a key finding to differentiate PB from ACC in the current classification.[1,2]

ACC and neuroendocrine tumor (NET) might be confused histologically; especially NETs with abundant eosinophilic (oncocytic) cytoplasm or acinar arrangement might be challenging. In general, single prominent nucleoli, chromophilic or granular eosinophilic cytoplasm, basal nuclear polarization, abundant acinar formations, no or minimal fibrotic stroma within neoplastic nodules, and an elevated mitotic rate favor a diagnosis of ACC rather than NET (see **Figs. 2** and **3**).[1,2] In addition, immunohistochemical labeling (acinar marker, trypsin; endocrine marker, chromogranin or synaptophysin) is helpful to distinguish these neoplasms. However, it should be noted that some NETs focally express acinar markers and, similarly, scattered individual cells (by definition less than 25% of the tumor cells) labeling for chromogranin A or synaptophysin are found in more than one-third of ACC cases.[5,8]

PANCREATOBLASTOMA

OVERVIEW

Although PB is an uncommon malignant epithelial neoplasm of the pancreas, it is the most frequent pancreatic neoplasm in childhood, with most occurring in the first decade of life.[2] Some cases have been reported in association with Beckwith-Wiedemann syndrome. PBs reveal multiple directions of differentiation and possess squamoid nests (**Figs. 4** and **5**).[9,10] Squamoid nests are regarded as a defining component of PB and are critical for establishing the diagnosis.[1,2] No gender predominance or preferential localization is seen. Patients most commonly are asymptomatic or present with nonspecific symptoms, such as abdominal pain, weight loss, or nausea. Jaundice is uncommon. An abdominal mass is often palpable. A quarter of patients have elevated serum AFP levels,[11] a marker that, when present, can be used to monitor the effectiveness of therapy.

GROSS FEATURES

PBs are usually large at presentation. The size ranges from 1.5 to 20.0 cm, with a mean of 10.0 cm.[1,2] Most are, at least partially, well-circumscribed solid masses. Sectioning reveals tan to yellowish, soft lobules separated by stromal bands. Some may contain cystic spaces owing to hemorrhagic necrosis and cystic degeneration, which appear as heterogeneous or multiloculated masses on radiological images. Congenital cases in association with Beckwith-Wiedemann syndrome may be predominantly cystic.[12] Infiltration of adjacent structures may occur.

MICROSCOPIC FEATURES

The tumors are composed of highly cellular lobules separated by fibrous bands (see **Fig. 4**). The neoplastic cells within the lobules usually show an organoid arrangement of acinar, solid, or trabecular formations akin to ACCs. It is important to keep in mind that the density and distribution of squamoid nests (see **Fig. 4**) vary by regions, as well as by neoplasms, and that it may be difficult

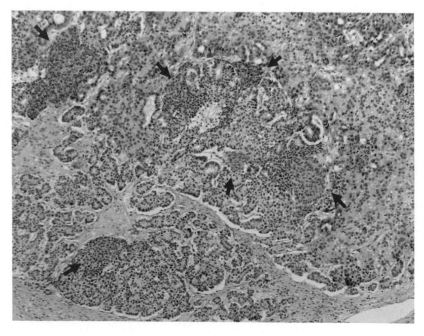

Fig. 4. Pancreatoblastoma. Tumor is composed of acinar structures and cellular lobules separated by fibrous bands. Squamoid nests (*arrows*) are scattered in the lobules (H&E stain, original magnification ×80).

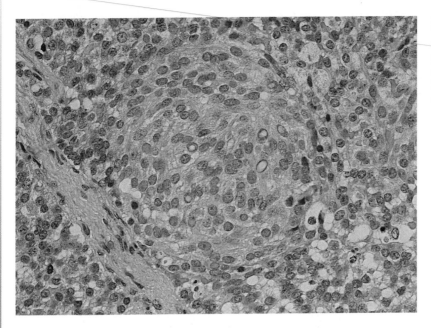

Fig. 5. Pancreatoblastoma. The squamoid nest contains a few cells with nuclear clearing (owing to intranuclear biotin) (H&E stain, original magnification ×400).

to detect them in small samples, such as biopsy or aspiration smears. These nests are composed of cells with eosinophilic to clear cytoplasm in formations varying from islands of epithelioid cells to whorled nests of spindled cells (see **Fig. 5**) and may demonstrate overt keratinization.[1,2] They lack cellular atypia, prominent nucleoli, and mitosis. Occasionally, nuclear clearing owing to the intranuclear accumulation of biotin may be seen (see **Fig. 5**).[13] In addition to the acinar component and squamous nests, a neuroendocrine component is detected, with the help of specific stains, in two-thirds of cases. A ductal/glandular component with mucin production or a primitive round-cell component is occasionally present and usually very focal.

Many cases show labeling for markers of acinar, ductal, and endocrine differentiation in the respective areas, although acinar differentiation is the most common and the predominant pattern in most cases. An abnormal (nuclear and cytoplasmic) immunolabeling pattern for the

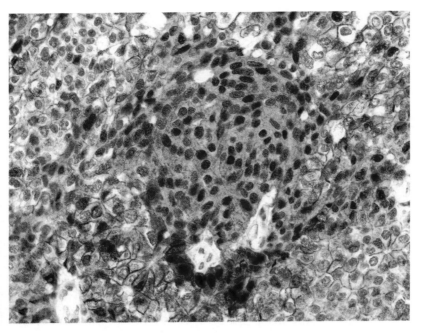

Fig. 6. Pancreatoblastoma. Abnormal (nuclear and cytoplasmic) labeling with β-catenin is seen in the squamoid nest (β-catenin immunohistochemical stain, original magnification ×400).

product of the β-catenin gene (**Fig. 6**) and overexpression of its target gene cyclin D1 is seen in most cases, usually in the squamoid nests.[14] Squamoid nests are also positive for epithelial membrane antigen. Immunohistochemical positivity for AFP has been detectable in cases with elevations in the serum levels of AFP.

DIFFERENTIAL DIAGNOSIS

When the mass is large and not clearly arising from the pancreas, common tumors of adjacent organs occurring in young children, including neuroblastoma, hepatoblastoma, and Wilms tumor must be considered. Among pancreatic neoplasms, ACC, SPN, and NET are in the differential diagnosis. However, none of these possess squamoid nests, and SPN and NET do not exhibit significant acinar differentiation. Expression of acinar enzymes, trypsin and chymotrypsin, along with endocrine and ductal markers, as well as an abnormal (nuclear and cytoplasmic) β-catenin expression, are diagnostic of PBs.

SOLID-PSEUDOPAPILLARY NEOPLASM

OVERVIEW

SPNs are unique neoplasms with uncertain direction of differentiation, occurring predominantly (90%) in adolescent girls and young women (mean, 28 years; range, 7 to 79 years).[1,2] They represent 0.9% to 2.7% of exocrine pancreatic neoplasms. There is no preferential localization within the pancreas. Rare cases arising in the retroperitoneum, mesocolon, and ovary have been reported.[1,15] SPNs are usually found incidentally on routine physical examination or imaging for another indication. If symptomatic, the symptoms are usually nonspecific. Jaundice is rare. Tumor rupture and hemoperitoneum related to abdominal trauma may be encountered.

GROSS FEATURES

SPNs usually form large, round, circumscribed solitary masses that are soft and friable. Their size ranges from 0.5 to 25.0 cm with a mean of 8.0 to 10.0 cm.[1,2] Sectioning reveals light brown to yellow solid tumor with areas of necrosis and remote or recent hemorrhage, sometimes in the form of cysts filled with blood (**Fig. 7**), which cause a heterogeneous appearance on radiological images. In large cystic neoplasms, residual solid areas are found only at the periphery of the tumor (see **Fig. 7**) and occasionally tumors mimic a pseudocyst. Small tumors tend to be more solid than larger examples. Some cases are firm and sclerotic. The tumors often compress adjacent structures rather than invading them.

MICROSCOPIC FEATURES

SPNs have a peculiar microscopic appearance. The growth pattern is heterogeneous, with

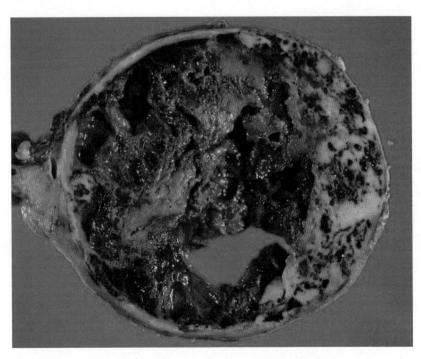

Fig. 7. Solid-pseudopapillary neoplasm. The tumor is an encapsulated neoplasm including marked hemorrhagic debris. Residual solid component is seen at the periphery (*right*).

a combination of solid, pseudopapillary, pseudo-glandular, and hemorrhagic-necrotic pseudocys-tic components in variable amounts. The solid component is composed of uniform, polygonal epithelioid cells admixed with thin-walled blood vessels. The preferential dyscohesiveness of the cells away from these vessels may lead to the highly distinctive arrangement of cells that is referred as "pseudopapillary," although it is not present in all cases. Fine-needle aspiration cytology can highlight the pattern of delicate branching vessels and loosely cohesive mono-morphic cells. There is no real gland formation. The cells have either eosinophilic or clear vacuo-lated cytoplasm with round to oval nuclei that have finely dispersed chromatin and often longitu-dinal grooves (**Fig. 8**). Bizarre nuclei may occasionally be seen. Intracytoplasmic or extra-cytoplasmic, diastase-resistant PAS-positive, eosinophilic globules are usually intermingled (see **Fig. 8**). Aggregates of foamy macrophages and cholesterol crystals are also present. Despite the well-circumscribed gross appearance, infiltra-tive edges entrapping acinar cells and islets is a common finding. Calcification and ossification may be seen in the associated hyalinized connective tissue or in the capsule. Vascular and perineural invasions are rare and mitotic rate is usually low.

Cytokeratins (CAM 5.2, AE1/AE3) are typically either negative or only very focal in SPNs. However, the neoplastic cells express vimentin and α-1 anti-trypsin diffusely and strongly. Other markers consistently expressed in SPN are CD10, CD56, progesterone receptor, and abnormal (nuclear and cytoplasmic) β-catenin.[16,17] Recently, C-kit (CD117) and FLI-1 expressions have been reported in a portion of SPNs.[18,19]

VARIANTS

SPN with apparent high-grade malignant transfor-mation is a recently described entity for highly aggressive SPNs showing diffuse solid growth patterns, as well as necrosis, increased cellular atypia, high nuclear to cytoplasmic ratio, and abundant mitoses (**Fig. 9**), or a sarcomatoid (spindle cell) carcinoma component.[2,20]

DIFFERENTIAL DIAGNOSIS

The differential diagnosis from ACC or PB is dis-cussed in the section on pancreatoblastomas. Histologic and cytologic appearances of SPN can also overlap with those of NET, but their char-acteristic clinical presentation, imaging features, and immunohistochemical features help distin-guish these neoplasms. Especially, abnormal (nuclear and cytoplasmic) β-catenin expression and no immunoreactivity for chromogranin A in SPNs are helpful.

PROGNOSIS

All 3 neoplasms reviewed in this article have more or less metastatic potential and most commonly

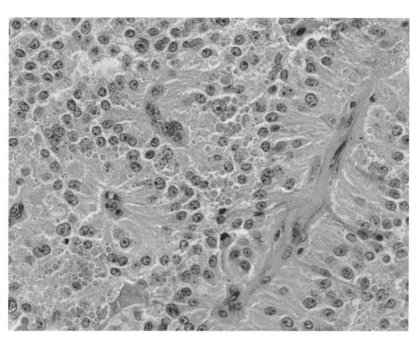

Fig. 8. Solid-pseudopapil-lary neoplasm. Degenerative pseudopapillae, charac-terized with loosely cohe-sive round to oval uniform cells surrounding delicate capillary-sized blood vessels, are seen. Eosinophilic hyalin globules are intermingled (H&E stain, original mag-nification ×400).

Fig. 9. High-grade malignant solid-pseudopapillary neoplasm. The tumor shows diffuse growth with increased cellularity, marked pleomorphism, high nuclear/cytoplasmic ratio, and many mitoses (*arrows*) (H&E stain, original magnification ×400).

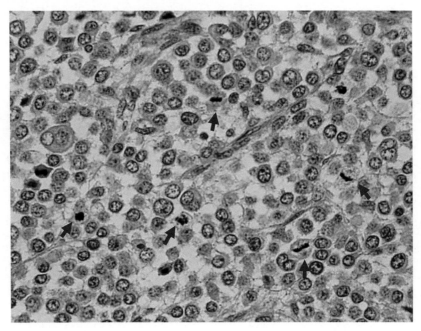

metastasize to regional lymph nodes and/or the liver. Metastases are found in 50% of patients with ACC, 17% to 35% of patients with PB, and 5% to 15% of patients with SPN at the time of presentation,[2] indicating their different biologic behavior.

Stage, thus resectability, is an important prognostic factor for all of them. In ACC and PB, patients with nonresectable disease usually do not survive beyond 5 years, but patients with surgically resectable disease have a favorable prognosis, with a 5-year survival of 25% to 50% and 65%, respectively.[2] In SPN, almost all cases are resectable and 85% to 95% of patients are cured after complete surgical resection.[2]

However, there are reports of long survival even in the presence of local spread, recurrences, or metastases after initial diagnosis and resection for all types, although the frequency is largely different by types (more frequent in SPN), which indicates that these neoplasms contain various malignant grades. However, no grading system that can predict outcome has been proposed for any of these neoplasms. Establishment of such a grading system would be helpful.

REFERENCES

1. Hruban RH, Pitman MB, Klimstra DS, editors. AFIP atlas of tumor pathology, fourth series, fascicle 6: tumors of the pancreas. Washington, DC: American Registry of Pathology; 2007. p. 23–304.

2. Bosman FT, Carneiro F, Hruban RH, et al, editors. WHO classification of tumours of the digestive system. Lyon (France): International Agency for Research on Cancer; 2010. p. 314–30.

3. Ban D, Shimada K, Sekine S, et al. Pancreatic ducts as an important route of tumor extension for acinar cell carcinoma of the pancreas. Am J Surg Pathol 2010;34:1025–36.

4. Morohoshi T, Kanda M, Horie A, et al. Immunocytochemical markers of uncommon pancreatic tumors. Acinar cell carcinoma, pancreatoblastoma, and solid cystic (papillary-cystic) tumor. Cancer 1987;59:739–47.

5. Ohike N, Kosmahl M, Klöppel G. Mixed acinar-endocrine carcinoma of the pancreas. A clinicopathological study and comparison with acinar-cell carcinoma. Virchows Arch 2004;445:231–5.

6. Basturk O, Zamboni G, Klimstra DS, et al. Intraductal and papillary variants of acinar cell carcinomas. Am J Surg Pathol 2007;31:363–70.

7. Klimstra DS, Rosai J, Heffess CS. Mixed acinar-endocrine carcinomas of the pancreas. Am J Surg Pathol 1994;18:765–78.

8. Ohike N, Morohoshi T. Pathological assessment of pancreatic endocrine tumors for metastatic potential and clinical prognosis. Endocr Pathol 2005;16: 33–40.

9. Becker WF. Pancreatoduodenectomy for carcinoma of the pancreas in an infant: report of a case. Ann Surg 1957;145:864–72.

10. Horie A, Yano Y, Kotoo Y, et al. Morphogenesis of pancreatoblastoma, infantile carcinoma of the pancreas: report of two cases. Cancer 1977;39: 247–54.

11. Morohoshi T, Sagawa F, Mitsuya T. Pancreatoblastoma with marked elevation of serum alpha-fetoprotein. An

autopsy case report with immunocytochemical study. Virchows Arch A Pathol Anat Histopathol 1990;416: 265–70.

12. Drut R, Jones MC. Congenital pancreatoblastoma in Beckwith-Wiedemann syndrome: an emerging association. Pediatr Pathol 1988;8:331–9.

13. Tanaka Y, Ijiri R, Yamanaka S, et al. Pancreatoblastoma: optically clear nuclei in squamoid corpuscles are rich in biotin. Mod Pathol 1998;11:945–9.

14. Tanaka Y, Kato K, Notohara K, et al. Significance of aberrant (cytoplasmic/nuclear) expression of beta-catenin in pancreatoblastoma. J Pathol 2003;199: 185–90.

15. Deshpande V, Oliva E, Young RH. Solid pseudopapillary neoplasm of the ovary: a report of 3 primary ovarian tumors resembling those of the pancreas. Am J Surg Pathol 2010;34:1514–20.

16. Notohara K, Hamazaki S, Tsukayama C, et al. Solid-pseudopapillary tumor of the pancreas: immunohistochemical localization of neuroendocrine markers and CD10. Am J Surg Pathol 2000;24: 1361–71.

17. Tanaka Y, Kato K, Notohara K, et al. Frequent beta-catenin mutation and cytoplasmic/nuclear accumulation in pancreatic solid-pseudopapillary neoplasm. Cancer Res 2001;61:8401–4.

18. Ohike N, Sato M, Hisayuki T, et al. Immunohistochemical analysis of nestin and c-kit and their significance in pancreatic tumors. Pathol Int 2007;57: 589–93.

19. Tiemann K, Kosmahl M, Ohlendorf J, et al. Solid pseudopapillary neoplasms of the pancreas are associated with FLI-1 expression, but not with EWS/FLI-1 translocation. Mod Pathol 2006;19:1409–13.

20. Tang LH, Aydin H, Brennan MF, et al. Clinically aggressive solid pseudopapillary tumors of the pancreas: a report of two cases with components of undifferentiated carcinoma and a comparative clinicopathologic analysis of 34 conventional cases. Am J Surg Pathol 2005;29:512–9.

CONUNDRUMS AND CAVEATS IN NEUROENDOCRINE TUMORS OF THE PANCREAS

Laura H. Tang, MD, PhD*, David S. Klimstra, MD

KEYWORDS

- Pancreas • Endocrine • Neuroendocrine • Neuroendocrine tumor • Neuroendocrine neoplasm
- Islet cell tumor • Somatostatin receptor • Chromogranin • Ki 67

ABSTRACT

Pancreatic neuroendocrine tumors (Pan-NETs) are the second most common epithelial neoplasm of the pancreas after ductal adenocarcinoma. They can be clinically defined as functional, nonfunctional, and hereditary. This review addresses typical and atypical pathologic features of Pan-NETs, with a focus on practical issues involved in differential diagnosis, immunohistochemical work-up, intraoperative frozen section interpretation, sources of diagnostic errors, and classification. The diagnosis of a Pan-NET requires analysis of all available clinical and radiographic information and pathologic characteristics of the tumor, and it is crucial to understand the clinical impact of the pathologic interpretation.

OVERVIEW

Pancreatic neuroendocrine tumors (Pan-NETs) were initially described a century ago by Nicholls[1] and currently represent the second most common epithelial neoplasm after ductal adenocarcinoma of the pancreas.[2] Given the increased accessibility and sensitivity of imaging modalities, Pan-NETs are no longer considered rare neoplasms and account for 1% to 2% of pancreatic tumors. Because most Pan-NETs initially comprised benign symptomatic insulin-producing tumors (insulinomas), they were erroneously considered a benign group of neoplasm. In the past 3 decades, however, it has become apparent that 50% or more Pan-NETs are nonfunctional, and they are a heterogeneous group of tumors with often unpredictable and varying degrees of malignancy. As many as 50% to 80% Pan-NETs are associated with synchronous or metachronous metastatic disease.[3] Knowledge of functional Pan-NETs has evolved from insulinoma to almost a dozen other diverse hormone-secreting tumors. These individual lesions may have specific clinical, pathologic, and genetic associations, including multiple endocrine neoplasia type 1 (MEN-1), tuberouse sclerosis, and von Hippel-Lindau (vHL) syndromes. Thus, the entity of Pan-NET represents a diverse group of heterogeneous neoplasms; combined clinical and pathologic assessment is required to further identify their genetic basis for neoplasia and to define their specific clinical behavior. The nonfunctional tumors require further elucidation to characterize their diverse pathogenesis and to predict outcome with potential biomarkers and molecular signatures.

The histopathologic diagnosis of a typical Pan-NET in a surgical specimen is usually straightforward, particularly if clinical correlation (symptoms, imaging data, or tumor biomarker levels) is

Department of Pathology, Memorial Sloan-Kettering Cancer Center, 1275 York Avenue, New York, NY 10065, USA
* Corresponding author.
E-mail address: tangl@mskcc.org

Surgical Pathology 4 (2011) 589–624
doi:10.1016/j.path.2011.03.003
1875-9181/11/$ – see front matter © 2011 Elsevier Inc. All rights reserved.

surgpath.theclinics.com

Key Features
OF PAN-NET

Clinical and Radiographic

- Defined as functional, nonfunctional, hereditary (not always apparent)
- Any age (a decade younger than mean onset age of ductal carcinoma)
- Jaundice uncommon
- Radiographically well circumscribed and hypervascular enhancing on contrast CT
- Majority PET negative (particularly in low-grade tumors)
- Octreoscan avid in approximately 80%

Gross Pathology

- Well circumscribed (at least for small lesions)
- Yellow-tan or hemorrhagic in color
- Relatively homogenous in appearance (occasionally cystic and degenerative)
- Soft and fleshy in consistency (occasionally sclerotic)
- Pancreatic duct obstruction/obliteration is unusual.

Histopathology

- Organoid pattern with nests, trabecular, gyriform, or hyaline vascular architecture
- Abundant and delicate vasculature
- Abundant eosinophilic/amphophilic cytoplasm without a distinct cell membrane border
- Uniform nuclei and stippled chromatin pattern, but nuclear pleomorphism can occur.
- Most (approximately 60%) are low grade with mitotic activity of <2/50 high-power fields (HPFs).
- Positive immunoreactivity for cytokeratin and synaptophysin supports the diagnosis (if hematoxylin-eosin stain is suboptimal).
- Ki-67 is helpful to assess tumor grade when evaluation of mitosis is difficult.
- The pathologic diagnosis of Pan-NET must distinguish a well-differentiated tumor (low or intermediate grade) from a poorly differentiated NE carcinoma (only high grade).
- Poorly differentiated NE carcinoma of the pancreas is a rare entity and may present as a component admixed acinar cell carcinoma or ductal carcinoma.
- The diagnosis of Pan-NET in a pancreatic or liver biopsy and in intraoperative frozen sections can be challenging; the differential diagnosis includes other primary neoplasms of the pancreas and the liver as well as metastatic tumors.

Specific Features of Functional or Syndromic Pan-NETs

- Symptoms are related to specific bioactive agents secreted by tumor.
- Some tumors may be radiographically occult.
- Histopathology or immunohistochemical findings alone cannot differentiate between functional and nonfunctional lesions.
- Elevated plasma biomarkers are most sensitive in diagnosis.
- Gross multicentricity is usually evident in hereditary settings (MEN-1 and vHL).
- Microadenomas or abnormal islets are identifiable in hereditary settings (MEN-1 and vHL).

available. Difficulties, however, have arisen with increasing volume of small and suboptimal biopsy specimens of nonfunctional Pan-NETs from either primary or metastatic sites. Under such circumstances, the differential diagnosis can be wide and the pathologic interpretation challenging. This is relevant with recent reorganization of diverse morphologic variants of Pan-NETs.[4–6]

Several different classification and staging systems have been proposed for Pan-NETs, and there is continuous debate regarding the determination of tumor grade and the optimal markers for prediction of outcome. Each of the different systems has both strengths and weaknesses and none has achieved universal acceptance.[7–10]

It is thus important to understand the specific parameters required to report Pan-NETs to accumulate practical and accurate pathologic information for the development of an ideal and accurate classification system.[11]

This review addresses key pathologic features as well as relevant clinical and molecular characteristics of Pan-PET with a focus on practical issues involved in differential diagnosis in biopsies and difficult cases, immunohistochemical work-up, and classification issues.

RADIOGRAPHIC FEATURES

Most Pan-NETs have a solid and enhancing appearance on contrast CT scans due to their rich vascularity (**Fig. 1**). In contrast to ductal carcinomas, Pan-PETs rarely cause obstruction and secondary dilatation of pancreatic or biliary ducts, although this may be a feature of a subset of nonfunctional lesions that may grow to a larger size before detection. Large tumors extend to peripancreatic soft tissue, the retroperitoneum, or adjacent organs in an expansile fashion (**Fig. 2**). A small percentage of Pan-NETs demonstrate cystic change that may sometimes be extensive. Thus, the distinction of an entirely cystic Pan-NET from cystic ductal neoplasms may be difficult on imaging studies. Low-grade Pan-NETs are usually positron emission tomography (PET) negative and the identification of a PET avid tumor suggests the likelihood of a higher grade and clinically more aggressive tumor (see Key Features box). Most Pan-NETs express somatostatin types 2 and 5 receptors; thus, somatostatin receptor scintigraphy (Octreoscan [indium 111 octreotide, a somatostatin analog]) is positive in up to 80% tumors although a negative scan does not exclude a neuroendocrine (NE) tumor.[12,13] A negative Octreoscan in an individual with a proved Pan-NET is suggestive of a high grade or aggressive tumor because such lesions often do not express somatostatin receptors.[14] The signal on scintigraphy reflects the density of somatostatin receptor in tumor cells, and it is not necessarily associated with actual tumor size. An Octreoscan is helpful in the identification of distant metastases or locating an occult primary in individuals who present with metastatic disease in the absence of an apparent pancreatic lesion (see **Fig. 2**C).

GROSS PATHOLOGIC FEATURES

Pan-NETs arise in the tail of pancreas (60%) more commonly than in the head and body. Functional tumors are typically smaller than nonfunctional lesions because the presence of hormonal-related symptoms leads to an earlier clinical presentation. Most Pan-NETs are sharply demarcated from the adjacent pancreatic parenchyma or even encapsulated; they are usually homogeneous and fleshy in consistency although some can be firm and sclerotic and are yellow to red-tan in color (**Fig. 3**). Large Pan-NETs are often present as bosselated or multinodular lesions, which can demonstrate gross invasion into peripancreatic tissues, mesentery, or adjacent organs (eg, spleen, kidney, stomach, duodenum, and colon) (see **Fig. 2**). Vascular invasion may be grossly evident, particularly in a distal pancreatic mass where splenic venous invasion may occur.

Partially cystic tumors are usually secondary to degenerative changes and are not uncommon. The presence of extensive cystic change in a Pan-NET, however, may generate both radiographic and gross pathologic confusion given its resemblance to non-NE cystic pancreatic neoplasms (**Fig. 4**). In most cases, cystic Pan-NETs have a solitary locule surrounded by a rim of neoplastic parenchyma that is often separated from the adjacent pancreas by a fibrous pseudocapsule.[15]

MICROSCOPIC FEATURES

CHARACTERISTIC HISTOPATHOLOGIC FEATURES OF WELL-DIFFERENTIATED PAN-NETS

Microscopically, most Pan-NETs are easily recognized by one or more of the characteristic organoid patterns with nested, trabecular, gyriform, or hyaline vascular architecture (**Fig. 5**; Differential Diagnosis Table). Clusters of neoplastic cells are usually separated by abundant and delicate vessels lined by inconspicuous endothelial cells. In addition, glandular/lumen formation may occur, usually within a large nest of cells,

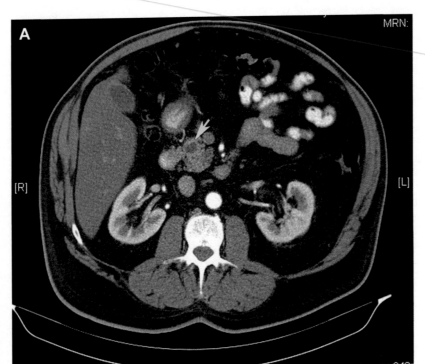

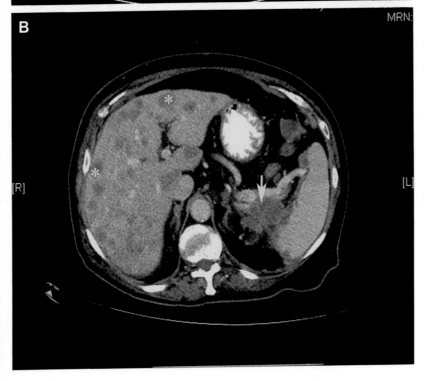

Fig. 1. Identification of Pan-NETs on CT scans. (*A*) A small enhancing lesion is localized in the head of the pancreas (*arrow*). (*B*) An enhancing tumor is present in the tail of the pancreas (*arrow*). Numerous metastatic lesions are evident in the liver (*).

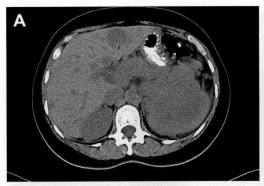

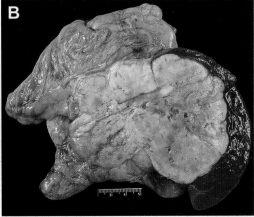

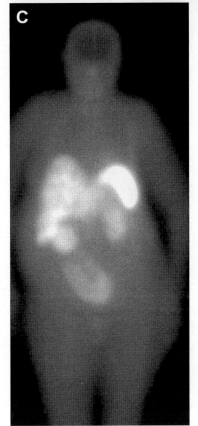

Fig. 2. Pan-NET with extensive invasion to adjacent structures. (*A*) CT scan of a Pan-NET demonstrating a large and expansile lesion with invasion of adjacent structures, including the colonic mesentery and spleen, and liver metastasis. (*B*) The corresponding gross specimen demonstrating tumor invasion into the peripancreatic soft tissue, spleen, and mesentery of colon. (*C*) Octreoscan demonstrating tumor avidity in both primary and metastatic lesions, which is indicative of somatostatin receptor overexpression.

imparting a cribriform pattern. Both perineural and vascular invasion can occur and are usually present in the nerves and vessels at the periphery of the tumor or within the pseudocapsule. Given the ample vasculature of Pan-NETs, vascular invasion in small vessels within the tumor should be interpreted with caution because the vessels may actually represent a component of the tumor and be intimately intermingled with the tumor cells (**Fig. 6**). In contrast to ductal adenocarcinoma, Pan-NETs, in general, do not involve the pancreatic duct; however, tumor extension into the pancreatic ducts has been documented. Although most Pan-NETs are hypercellular and stroma poor, in some cases, collagen expansion, sometimes with amyloid deposition (especially in insulinomas),

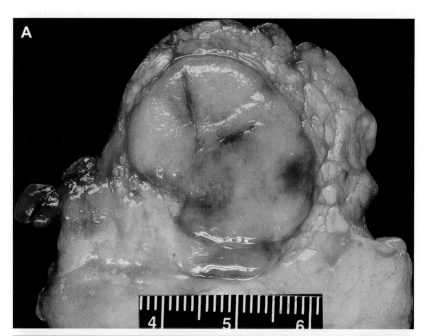

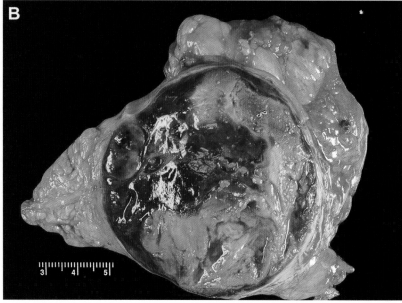

Fig. 3. Gross appearance of Pan-NETs. (*A*) A solid and well-circumscribed small (2.2-cm) tumor with a soft and fleshy consistency. (*B*) A large (6.5-cm) tumor with multifocal hemorrhage and degenerative changes.

between tumor nests, or around vessels can produce densely hyalinized stroma; and the neoplastic cells are compressed within the stroma and become a minor component of the tumor. This phenomenon, particularly in small biopsies, may create an impression that reminiscent of a benign vascular lesion (**Fig. 7A**). Also, a portion of Pan-NETs may present with vascular ectasia leaving only rare and small tumor nests around the thin-walled vessels; however, this change is usually focal and unlikely to mislead to an interpretation of a vascular lesion, at least

Fig. 4. Cystic Pan-NET. (*A*) Partial cystic degeneration of a Pan-NET. (*B*) A completely cystic Pan-NET with a thick fibrous capsule.

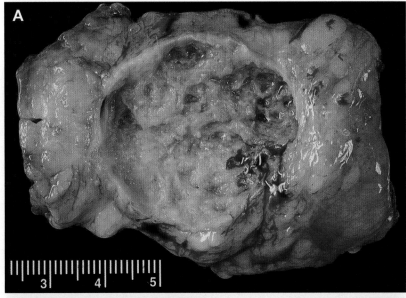

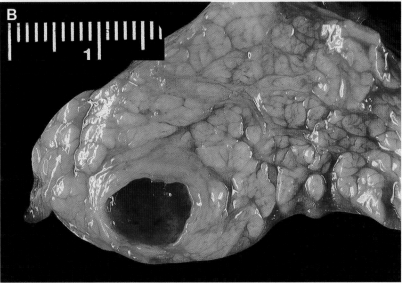

not in a surgically resected specimen (see **Fig. 7**B).

The tumor cells usually have abundant eosinophilic or amphophilic cytoplasm and, although they may vary in size, are usually polygonal in shape and without distinct cell borders (**Fig. 8**A, B). The tumor nucleus is either centrally or peripherally located but occasionally an extreme peripheral

nuclear location results in a plasmacytoid appearance (**Fig. 8**C). Cytoplasmic hyaline globules are uncommon but if present produce an appearance that resembles that of a solid pseudopapillary neoplasm (discussed later).

Typical nuclear features in Pan-NET are common to those of well-differentiated NETs at other sites of the gastrointestinal tract. The nuclei

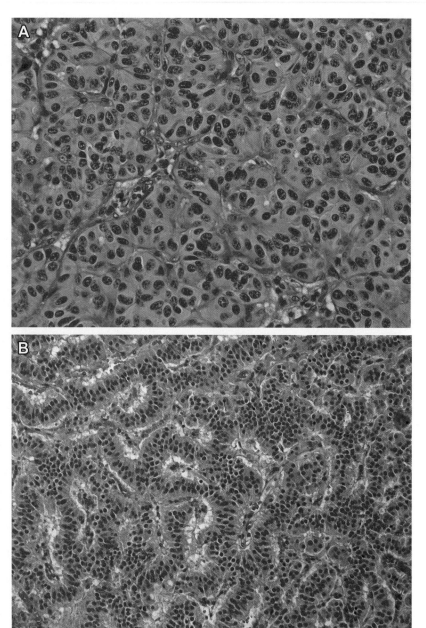

Fig. 5. Common histologic patterns of Pan-NET. (*A*) Nested pattern with tumor cells encircled by delicate vasculature. (*B*) Trabecular pattern with ribbons of tumor cells separated by delicate vasculature.

are usually round and uniform in size and shape and characteristically have a finely stippled salt-and-pepper appearance and are better appreciated in well-fixed tissue (eg, at the periphery of tumor sections or in smaller sections) (**Fig. 9**). Nuclei with coarsely clumped chromatin, open chromatin, or hyperchromatia are usually seen in poorly preserved tissue and are not necessarily associated with unfavorable pathologic features. Nucleoli of Pan-NETs are usually inconspicuous.

Most Pan-NETs have mitotic rate in the range of less than 2 mitoses per 50 HPFs. Because tumors

Fig. 5. (*C*) Gyriform pattern with elongated tumor cells arranged in folding trabeculae. (*D*) Hyaline vascular pattern with thickened vascular walls.

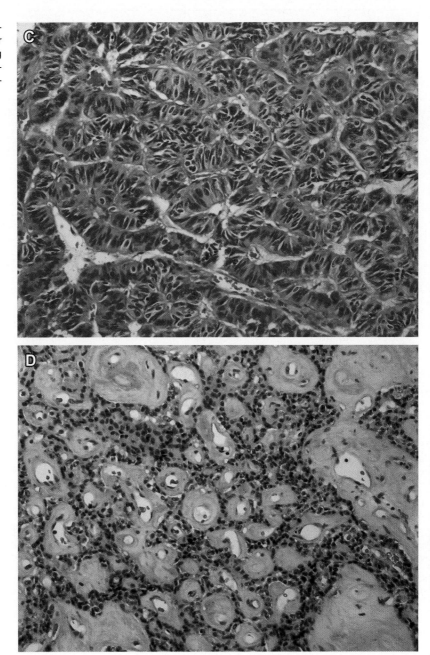

with modest increase in mitotic activity ($\geq$2/50 HPFs) are associated with more frequent recurrence or metastasis,[3,16] a thorough assessment of mitotic activity at high microscopic power in multiple fields is necessary; and this information should be included in the pathology report. Well-differentiated Pan-NETs with mitoses in the range of 10 to 20 mitoses per 10 HPFs are rare; and they may be seen in association with a dominant component of a typically low-grade tumor (**Fig. 10**). When mitotic activity of a tumor exceeds 20 mitoses per 10 HPFs, the interpretation of a high-grade NE

Differential Diagnosis
HISTOLOGIC FEATURES

	Well-Differentiated Pan-NET	Solid and Pseudopapillary Tumor	Acinar Cell Carcinoma/ Pancreablastoma	High-Grade Neuroendocrine Carcinoma
Border	Circumscribed/ encapsulated	Interdigitating with pancreatic parenchyma	Circumscribed/ encapsulated	Infiltrative
Pattern	Organoid/nested/ Trabecular/ hyaline vascular/ gyriform Delicate vasculature	Pseudopapillae Solid/cystic Blood lakes	Solid and nested Acinar arrangement Squamoid nests in pancreatoblastoma	Solid or infiltrative Geographic necrosis
Stroma	Minimal in most Hyalinization in some	Perivascular myxoid stroma	Minimal within tumor nodules	Minimal within tumor nodules
Inter/intra cellular features	Abundant cytoplasm (granular/ plasmacytoid/ clear/oncocytic) Indistinct cell border	Hyaline globules Cytoplasmic vacuolization Foam cells	Abundant eosinophilic cytoplasm Apical cytoplasmic granules	Minimal cytoplasm (small cell carcinoma) Moderate amount cytoplasm (large cell carcinoma)
Nuclei	Round Stippled Low-proliferation	Round or oval Grooved Low to non proliferation	Basal nuclear palisading Uniformed but atypical Prominent nucleoli Identifiable mitoses	Hyperchromatic Nucleoli: no in small cell carcinoma Nucleoli: yes in large cell carcinoma Frequent mitoses
Typical Immuno Profile	Cam 5.2+ Synaptophysin+ (diffusely) Chromogranin±	Cam 5.2− (or focal) Vimentin+ β-catinin+ (nuclear) CD10+	CK+ Trypsin+ Chymotrypsin+ Chromogranin± (focal) Synaptophysin± (focal)	CK+ Chromogranin+ (patchy or diffuse) Synaptophysin+ (patchy or diffuse) Ki-67 + >70% in most

	Unusual Ductal Carcinoma	Met Renal Cell Carcinoma	Pheochromocytoma	Angiomyolipoma (PEComa)
Border	Infiltrative	Usually circumscribed	Circumscribed	Circumscribed
Pattern	Solid/diffuse/ squamoid	Solid/cystic/ diffuse	Organoid	Loosely cohesive Epithelioid or spindle
Stroma	Desmoplasia	Minimal	Minimal	With large abnormal vessels Minimal fat component
Inter/intra cellular features	Intracellular mucin	Clear or granular cytoplasm	Abundant amphophilic granular cytoplasm	Clear (glycogen) or eosinophilic cytoplasm Perinuclear cytoplasmic condensation Indistinct cell border
Nuclei	Atypical Nucleoli± Proliferative	Atypical Nucleoli ± Proliferative	Large, may be pleomorphic Prominent nucleoli Non- to low proliferation	Eccentric in location Irregular nuclear membrane Non- to low proliferation
Typical Immuno Profile	CK+ mCEA+ MUC1+ p53+/SMAD4− (in 50%–60%)	CK− CA-IX+ CD10+	CK− Chromogranin+ S100+ (sustentacular cells)	CK− HMB45+

Fig. 6. Vascular invasion in Pan-NET. (*A*) Vascular invasion by a nest of tumor cells. (*B*) Pseudo-vascular invasion with neoplastic cells comprassing against the intratumoral vascular walls.

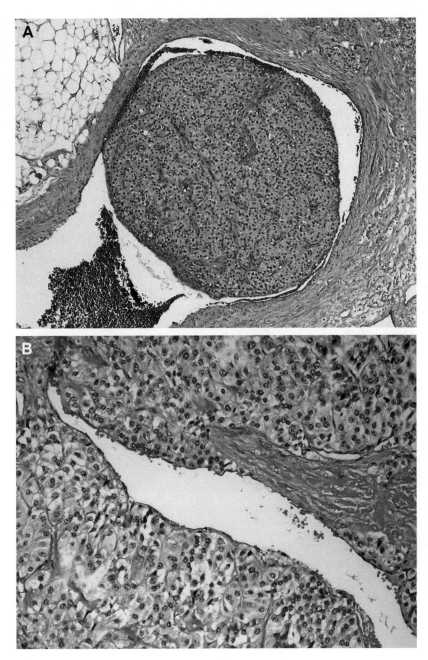

carcinoma should be entertained, particularly when there is no low-grade Pan-NET component or the tumor is admixed with a component of conventional ductal carcinoma (discussed later). Necrosis is not typically identified in smaller Pan-NETs (<2 cm).

When present, large foci of necrosis in well-differentiated Pan-NETs are usually infarct-like and probably represent an association with tumor trauma or a secondary event of ischemia due to occlusion of a large tumor feeding vessels. This

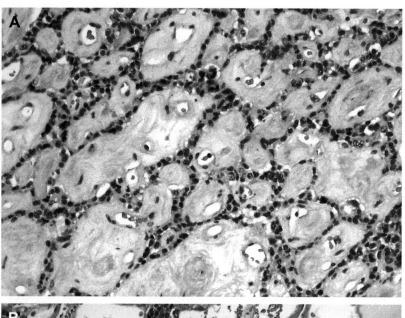

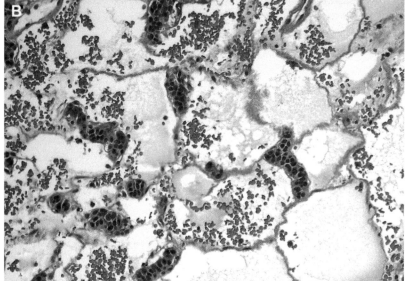

Fig. 7. Prominent hyaline vascular pattern of Pan-NET. (*A*) Vascular wall hyalinization dominating the architecture of the lesion with a minor component of linear tumor cells compressed between hyalinized vessels. (*B*) Thin-walled and ectatic vessels as a component of Pan-NET with scant tumor cells scattered between the vessels.

type of necrosis is usually confluent with architectural degenerations, which is characterized by loss of cohesive tumor architecture and the unity between tumor nests and vasculature. The tumor cells within the infarcted area reveal increased pleomorphism and hyperchromatic nuclei (**Fig. 11**). These alterations, however, are not indicative of a higher-grade tumor or a more pathologically aggressive neoplasm. Punctuate or microscopic foci of tumor necrosis in a well-differentiated

Fig. 8. Cytologic features of Pan-NET. (*A*) Typical cytologic features of a Pan-NET with abundant cytoplasm and stippled nuclei. (*B*) Pan-NET with eosinophilic and amphophilic cytoplasm. (*C*) A tumor with a plasmacytoid pattern secondary to excessive cytoplasm pushing the tumor nuclei to an eccentric location.

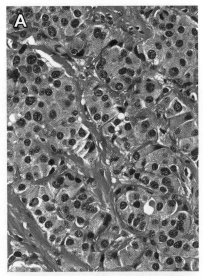

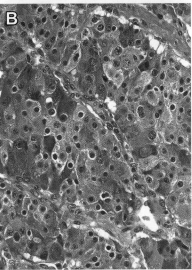

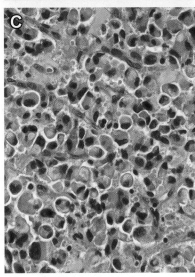

Pan-NET, on the contrary, occur in the center of the tumor nests and appear as aggregates of individual cells with partial or complete apoptosis (**Fig. 12**). The latter pattern of tumor necrosis is pathologically more important and is associated with tumor grade transformation.[17] Large and geographic tumor necrosis is commonly seen in poorly differentiated NE carcinoma (discussed later).

ATYPICAL MICROSCOPIC FEATURES OF WELL-DIFFERENTIATED PAN-NETS

Many morphologic variants, in addition to the classic patterns of Pan-NET (discussed previously), have been described. Oncocytic Pan-NETs are architecturally similar to conventional Pan-NETs but are composed of cells with abundant granular eosinophilic cytoplasm (**Fig. 13**A).[4] Clear cell change may also occur in Pan-NETs and is more common in Pan-NETs arising in individuals with vHL syndrome.[5,6] Neoplastic cells of Pan-NETs in vHL syndrome have abundant cytoplasm filled with numerous clear vesicles, resulting in foamy cytoplasm resembles that of sebaceous cells; intracellular lipid droplets have also been demonstrated (see **Fig. 13**B). Clear cell Pan-NETs should be distinguished from renal cell carcinoma metastatic to the pancreas, which is the most common metastatic malignancy in the pancreas (discussed later). Some Pan-NETs have marked nuclear atypia throughout the neoplasm and have been designated pleomorphic Pan-NETs.[6] Tumors with such features can be confused with high-grade neoplasms, such as ductal carcinomas or undifferentiated carcinomas. In contradistinction to its peculiar cytologic features, however, most pleomorphic Pan-NETs do not demonstrate an elevated mitotic rate or increased proliferative activity assessed by Ki-67, and the enlarged nuclei are accompanied by abundant cytoplasm (see **Fig. 13**C). Despite their worrisome appearance, no studies have demonstrated that pleomorphic Pan-NETs have a more aggressive biology than Pan-NETs with uniform nuclear morphology. Also reported is a variant of Pan-NETs with rhabdoid morphology. This variant characteristically has eccentrically located tumor nuclei and inclusion-like cytoplasm.

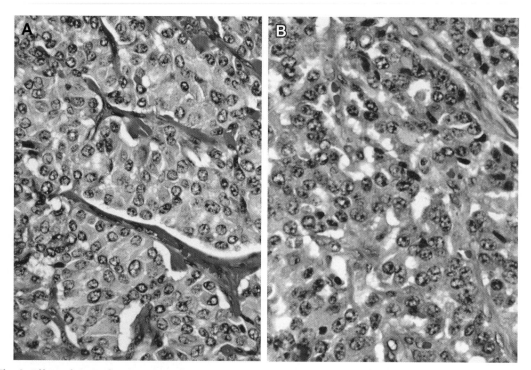

Fig. 9. Effect of tissue fixation on nuclear morphology of Pan-NET. Microphotographs from the same Pan-NET demonstrating (*A*) in well-fixed tissue with finely stippled nuclear characteristics and (*B*) in a suboptimally preserved portion of the tumor with nuclear overlapping and coarse chromatin.

POORLY DIFFERENTIATED NE CARCINOMA

This subtype of Pan-NET represents a rare entity and comprises at most 2% to 3% of pancreas NE neoplasms. Although designated NE because of their varying degree of NE differentiation, as demonstrated by positive immunoreactivity, often in a patchy or scant pattern, for generic NE markers (chromogranin, synaptophysin, or CD56), these tumors are more closely associated with conventional carcinomas than well-differentiated NE tumors of genuine NE lineage.[17] This hypothesis is supported by the fact that more than 75% of poorly differentiated NE carcinomas of the gastrointestinal tract and the pancreas are associated with an additional component of conventional carcinoma (either adenocarcinoma of squamous cell carcinoma[18]). The composites, adenocarcinoma–large cell high-grade NE carcinoma and squamous cell carcinoma–small cell high-grade NE carcinoma, have been documented as the most common histologic patterns. The tumors usually occur in adults and have a male predominance. Their clinical behavior is highly aggressive both locally and with widespread distant metastases. Functionality varies from nonfunctional status to ectopic production of numerous bioactive hormones with corticotropin the most common. Histopathologically, they have morphologic features, which are similar to those of high-grade NE carcinomas of other anatomic sites and comprise large cell and small cell types with high-grade cytologic features as well as an invariably high mitotic rate. Tumor necrosis is usually present as a geographic pattern (**Fig. 14**). Differential diagnosis includes nonpancreatic metastases, such as lung, ampulla, and other sites of the gastrointestinal tract, because a primary poorly differentiated NE carcinoma is rare.[19]

CYTOLOGY DIAGNOSIS

Pan-NETs are sometimes evaluated in cytology specimens performed via fine-needle aspiration (FNA) biopsy. The duct brushing cytology obtained

Fig. 10. Proliferative index (Ki-67) of Pan-NET. (*A*) Mitotic activity in a well-differentiated Pan-NET is usually inconspicuous and Ki-67 nuclear labeling usually in the range of 1% to 5% range. (*B*) Increased proliferative index seen in other areas of the same tumor from (*A*) with Ki-67 labeling up to approximately 30%.

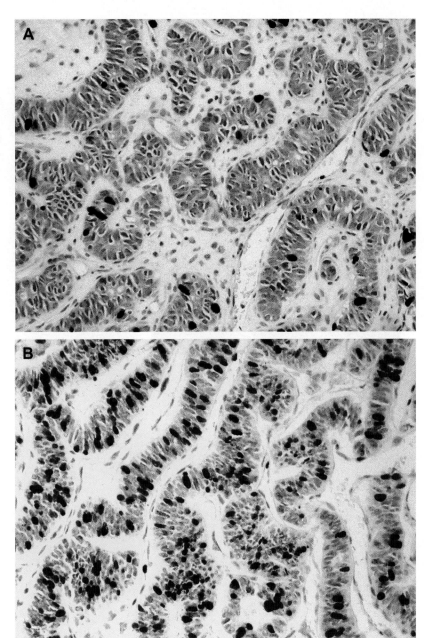

by endoscopy or endoscopic retrograde cholangiopancreatography has no diagnostic utility due to the lack of connection of the tumor with the pancreatic ductal system. CT-guided and endoscopic ultrasound FNA biopsy have equal sensitivity (94% to 95%) and specificity (100%) for the diagnosis of Pan-NET.[20]

Aspirate smears are usually hypercellular and composed of a monotonous population of small to medium-sized polygonal cells. The rich vascular

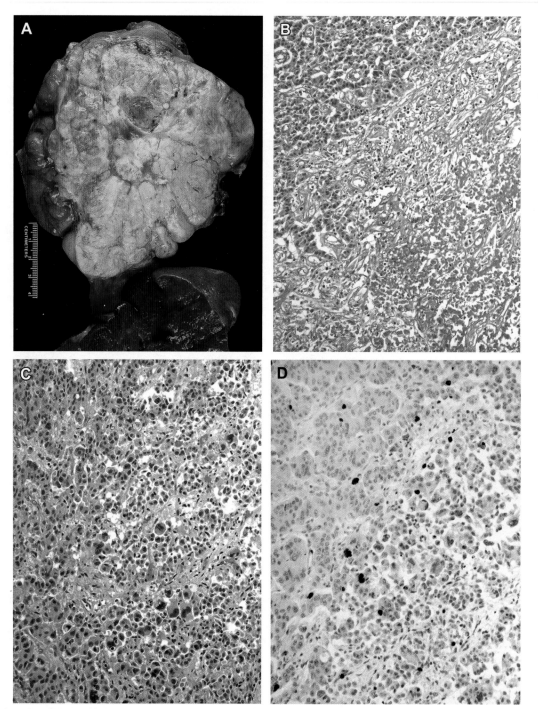

Fig. 11. Infarction-like necrosis in a large Pan-NET. (*A*) A gross photo of a 15-cm Pan-NET in the tail of the pancreas with a heterogeneous cut surface and areas of possible infarction. (*B*) The tumor exhibits microscopic infarction/necrosis with graduate loss of architecture and viable cellularity (*from upper left to lower right*). (*C*) Infarct-like necrosis is characterized by degeneration of both the nested architecture and individual cells with increased nuclear pleomorphism and hyperchromasia. (*D*) The infarcted tumor is not associated with increased mitotic activity or proliferative index (Ki-67).

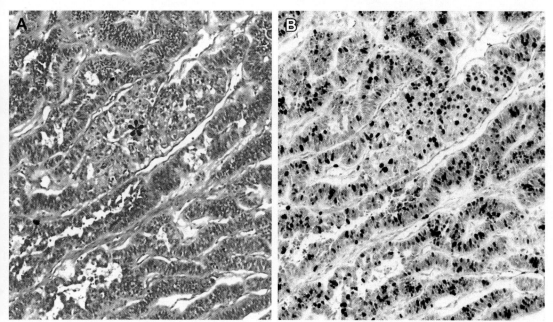

Fig. 12. Punctate/microscopic tumor necrosis in well-differentiated Pan-NET. (*A*) An intermediate-grade and well-differentiated Pan-NET with punctuate tumor necrosis characterized by a collection of individual cell apoptosis/necrosis (*). (*B*) Evidence of a higher tumor grade in area with tumor necrosis demonstrated by markedly increased Ki-67 proliferative index.

network of Pan-NETs typically produces a bloody background on cytology smears. The cells are mostly noncohesive or loosely cohesive and arranged as individual cells or in small to medium-sized groups (**Fig. 15**), which occasionally form rosettes. The cells have round nuclei, which have evenly distributed chromatin and are generally stippled. Nuclear atypia is variable, but in the majority of Pan-NETs, the nuclei are bland and uniform. The cytoplasm is relatively scant and usually dense and eccentric, yielding a plasmacytoid appearance, which is best appreciated in single cells. Mitotic figures are uncommon but may occasionally be seen. As on histology, the degree of nuclear atypia cannot be used to grade a Pan-NET or predict the outcome of the Pan-NET. Thus, a cytologic diagnosis should specify a well-differentiated Pan-NET without further grading unless there is evidence for features of possible poorly differentiated NE carcinoma in the differential diagnosis. Under such circumstances, a Ki-67 immunostain is most helpful; and greater than 50% nuclear labeling combined with morphologic features and easily identifiable mitoses enables an interpretation of a poorly differentiated NE carcinoma.

Given the characteristic cytologic features of most aspirates, immunocytochemical confirmation of the diagnosis is not always necessary. In difficult cases, confirmatory immunohistochemistry with chromogranin and/or synaptophysin can be performed either on destained smears or on formalin-fixed cell block preparations. Caution should be taken in the presence of ample amphophilic cytoplasm and prominent nucleoli, which could represent a peripancreatic pheochromocytoma/paraganglioma (**Fig. 16**). In such situations, it is prudent to perform a cytokeratin stain to confirm the nonepithelial nature of the tumor. Failure to recognize this entity may result in significant clinical consequences (eg, hypertensive crisis during the operation).

INTRAOPERATIVE FROZEN SECTION DIAGNOSIS

Intraoperative frozen sections may be performed to confirm the diagnosis of a Pan-NET, if the imaging studies are not conclusive and a diagnosis has not been previously confirmed via a biopsy or an aspiration, especially when a small or radiographically occult functional Pan-NET is suspected. It is not possible, however, by frozen section analysis to determine whether a given

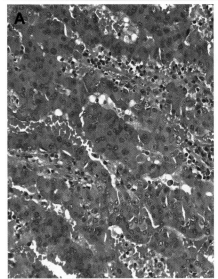

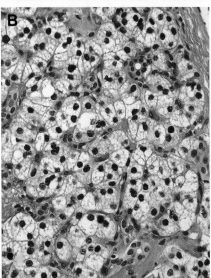

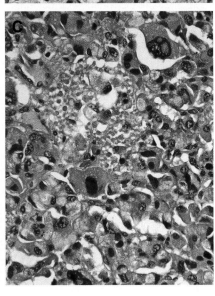

Fig. 13. Unusual patterns of well-differentiated Pan-NET. (*A*) Oncocytic variant with ample eosinophilic and granular cytoplasm. (*B*) Clear cell variant with foamy cytoplasm containing lipid droplets. (*C*) Pleomorphic variant with marked cytologic atypia and nuclear megaly.

Pan-NET is functional or nonfunctional. Preoperative and perioperative portal venous sampling of insulin has been used as an option in the localization of the symptomatic and radiographically occult insulinomas to specific regions of the pancreas.[21] If the diagnosis of Pan-NET is expected, based on clinical findings (eg, a hormone-related syndrome), the typical architectural and cytologic features are generally sufficient to confirm the diagnosis on frozen section. Several other primary pancreatic neoplasms, however, share the solid and hypercellular appearance of most Pan-NETs (discussed later) and may be difficult to distinguish from a Pan-NET at frozen section. The situation is pertinent and relatively common when dealing with a nonfunctional Pan-NET (**Fig. 17**). When a biopsy of liver metastasis is submitted for frozen section assessment without a prior diagnosis of a primary tumor, it is crucial to distinguish well-differentiated NETs from other metastatic carcinomas because it is surgical practice to proceed with resection of a primary Pan-NET even in the presence of documented hepatic or localized metastatic disease. On the contrary, a resection of primary ductal carcinoma in the presence of metastatic disease would be clinically contraindicated because these patients should receive chemotherapy as opposed to resection as the first-line of therapy.

DIFFERENTIAL DIAGNOSIS

As in any differential diagnostic work-up process, the most important strategy in Pan-NETs is to initially include all potential pathologic entities. This approach obviates omission of relevant pathologic entities that might occur based on misleading clinical information, illusory morphologic features, or a deceptive immunoprofile. The exclusion of specific alternative neoplastic processes is just as clinically relevant as the confirmation of the final diagnosis. Diagnosis of a Pan-NET in a surgically resected specimen is not difficult because both architectural and cytologic features (discussed previously) are usually better appreciated. Pan-NET in a pancreatic biopsy accompanied with or without an FNA, however, can be challenging. The judicious evaluation of available clinical and radiographic information, if provided, should be prudently used to support a final pathologic interpretation. Key

Fig. 14. Poorly differentiated (high-grade) NE
carcinoma of pancreas.
(*A*) High-grade NE carcinoma with a large area
of geographic necrosis
(*). (*B*) Combined ductal
(*left*) and high-grade NE
carcinoma (*right*).

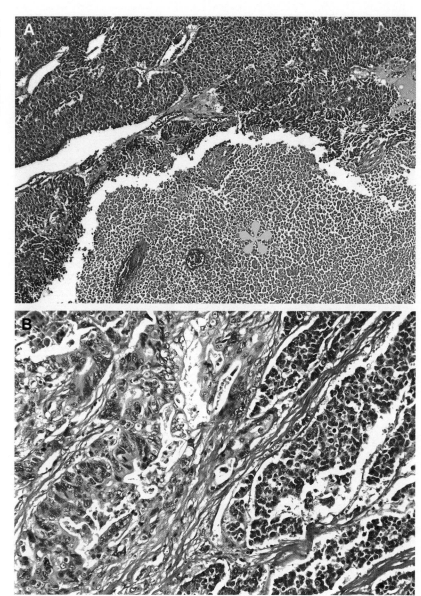

elements in the differential diagnosis include several pancreatic/peripancreatic primary tumors and other tumors commonly metastatic to the pancreas (see Differential Diagnosis of Pan-NET in a Pancreatic Specimen). The key pathologic features are detailed in the Differential Diagnosis table earlier in this article based on histology and representative microscopic photos that delineate key histologic features of the individual conditions are shown in **Figs. 18–21**.

Given a relatively high incidence of metastasis (50% to 80%), Pan-NET is more commonly seen in liver biopsies or extrapancreatic tissue in pathology practice. In liver biopsies, the rational diagnostic approach to a metastatic Pan-NET should include

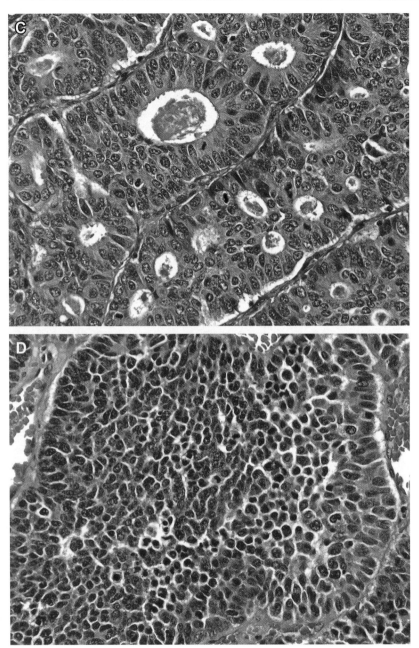

Fig. 14. (*C*) Large cell variant of high-grade NE carcinoma with moderate abundant eosinophilic cytoplasm, coarse chromatin and conspicuous nucleoli. (*D*) Small cell variant of high-grade NE carcinoma with minimal cytoplasm, hyperchromatic nuclei, inconspicuous nucleoli, and nuclear molding.

1. Exclusion of primary hepatic neoplasms (eg, hepatocellular carcinoma, peripheral cholangiocarcinoma, and, rarely, angiolipoma)
2. Consideration of metastatic well-differentiated NET of the gastrointestinal tract (eg, small bowel [most common], rectum, stomach, and appendix); atypical carcinoid of lung and medullary thyroid carcinoma
3. Elimination of other metastatic malignancies, which may imitate morphologic features of a well-differentiated NET (eg, pancreatic acinar cell carcinoma, renal cell carcinoma, adrenal cortical carcinoma, small cell or large cell NE carcinomas, solid variant of breast ductal carcinoma). See box, Differential Diagnosis of Pan-NET in Liver Biopsy.

Fig. 15. Well-differentiated NET on cytology smear from FNA. (*A*) Papanicolaou stain reveals a group of Pan-NET cells attached to a delicate vascular structure in a loosely cohesive fashion; the tumor cells have uniform nuclei and fine and slightly stippled chromatin. (*B*) Hematoxylin-eosin stain demonstrates neoplastic cells with abundant granular cytoplasm and eccentric nuclei yielding a plasmacytoid appearance. (*C*) A synaptophysin immunostain shows diffuse positive reactivity in tumor cells.

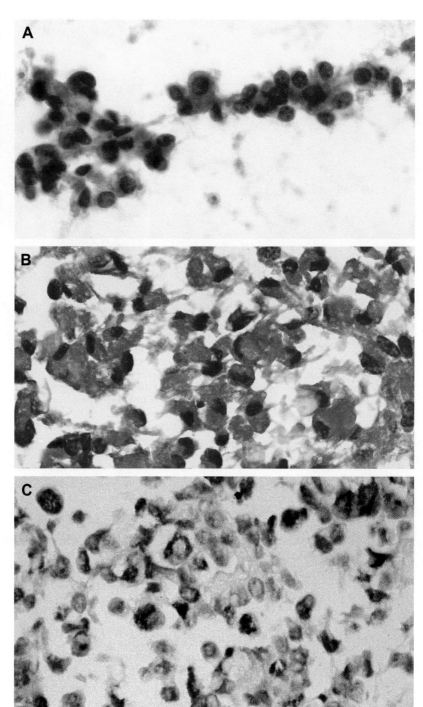

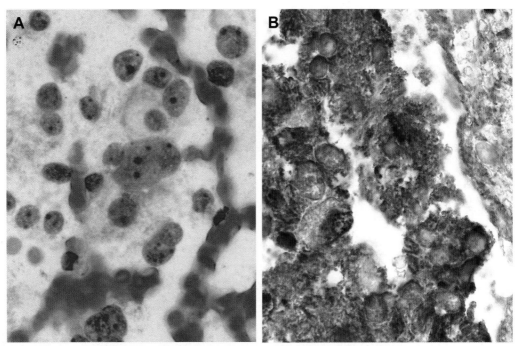

Fig. 16. Peripancreatic pheochromocytoma on cytology smear from FNA. (*A*) Papanicolaou stain reveals tumor cells with large nuclei, stippled chromatin, and conspicuous nucleloi. The granular cytoplasm is attached in some and stripped away in others resulting in naked nuclei appearance. (*B*) Immunostain of chromogranin is diffusely positive in tumor cells; a cytokeratin stain was not performed on cytology specimen, and was negative on resection specimen (not shown).

△△ Differential Diagnosis OF Pan-NET IN LIVER BIOPSY

1. Hepatocellular carcinoma

2. Peripheral cholangiocarcinoma

3. Primary angiomyolipoma

4. Metastatic nonpancreatic NETs

   A. Carcinoid tumors of gastrointestinal tract

   B. Atypical carcinoid tumor of lung

   C. Medullary thyroid carcinoma

   D. High-grade NE carcinoma of lung or other sites

5. Common metastatic non-NET

   A. Metastatic melanoma

   B. Breast carcinoma

   C. Renal cell carcinoma

   D. Adrenal cortical carcinoma

   E. Acinar cell carcinoma

△△ Differential Diagnosis OF Pan-NET IN A PANCREATIC SPECIMEN

- Solid and pseudopapillary tumor

- Acinar cell carcinoma/pancreatoblastoma

- High-grade NE carcinoma and mixed high-grade NE carcinoma and acinar cell carcinoma

- Peripancreatic pheochromocytoma

- Unusual histologic pattern in a ductal adenocarcinoma

- Angiomyolipoma (or peripancreatic epithelioid cell neoplasm [PEComa])

- Metastatic tumors (most commonly seen in surgical or biopsy specimens)
  - Renal cell carcinoma
  - Melanoma

Fig. 17. Intraoperative diagnosis of a pancreatic neoplasm imitating a Pan-NET. (*A*) Typical Pan-NET with nested pattern, abundant cytoplasm and low nuclear grade. (*B*) Pancreatic adenocarcinoma with a solid and nested pattern and moderate nuclear atypia.

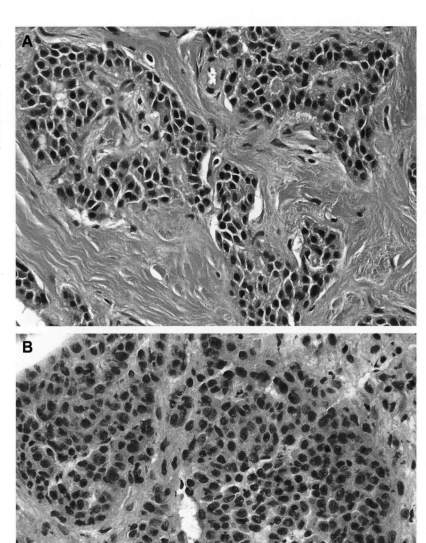

Representative microphotographs are provided in **Figs. 19–20**.

A critical difficulty often encountered in the diagnosis of a metastatic Pan-NET in liver biopsies is the lack of adequate clinical history and suboptimal biopsy material. The latter may comprise either inadequate tumor tissue or tissue with significant cautery or crush artifact. In some circumstances, tumor vasculature may present as governing morphology of the lesion, or tumor cells may be sloughed off from their nest leaving rare tumors cells attached to the encircling vasculature (see **Fig. 7**; **Fig. 21**). This phenomenon may, therefore, artifactually generate the appearance of a vascular lesion (eg, hepatic hemangioma). An immunostain for cytokeratin or synaptophysin,

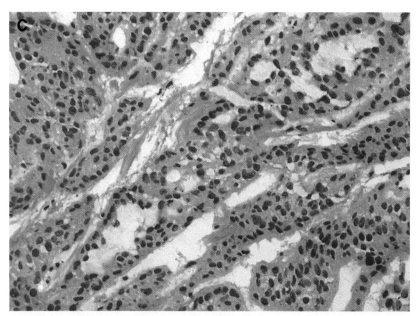

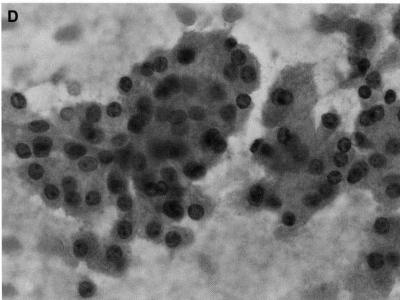

Fig. 17. (*C*) Frozen section of a solid and pseudopapillary tumor with cystic and vague papillary architecture and round to oval nuclei. (*D*) Solid and pseudopapillary tumor on cytology smear demonstrating small papillae with uniform nuclei and occasional nuclear grooves.

however, renders the diagnosis of a Pan-NET by identifying residual tumor cells within the vascular spaces (see **Fig. 21**). Tissue processing artifact either at the time of the procedure or in the histology laboratory may generate the impression of a high-grade NET or a poorly differentiated carcinoma of other entities. Under such circumstances, apart from documentation of NE differentiation by positive immunoreactivity for chromogranin and synaptophysin, an additional immunostain of Ki-67 is useful to demonstrate the low-grade nature of a well-differentiated Pan-NET (**Fig. 22**).

DIAGNOSIS

The diagnosis of a Pan-NET requires analysis of all available clinical and radiographic information and

Fig. 18. Differential diagnosis of Pan-NET occurring in the pancreas. (*A*) Solid component of a solid and pseudopapillary tumor with papillae formed around vascular cores. (*B*) Acinar cell carcinoma with acinar arrangement of the tumor cells, abundant granular and apically oriented cytoplasm, and atypical nuclear features.

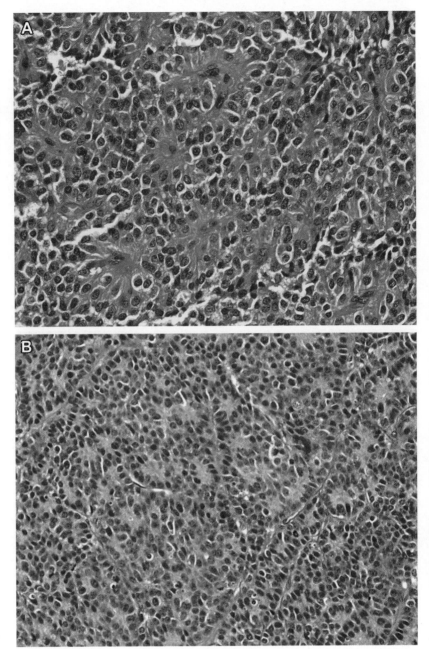

pathologic characteristics of the tumor.[15,22] In most situations, minimal ancillary pathologic work-up is required. The definitive diagnosis is confirmed by the morphology and positive immunoreactivity for cytokeratin (preferably Cam 5.2) and synaptophysin or chromogranin as well as negative immunoexpression of trypsin, chymotrypsin, and TTF1. The proliferative index assessed by Ki-67 immunoreactivity is usually in the range of 1% to 10%, and it may approach up to 40% in rare cases but only in foci within a predominantly low or intermediate tumor. This immunoprofile alone, however, does not distinguish a pancreatic primary from a gastrointestinal primary NET in a liver metastasis.

High-grade pancreatic NE carcinoma may arise in association with ductal adenocarcinoma as a composite carcinoma or it may be intimately

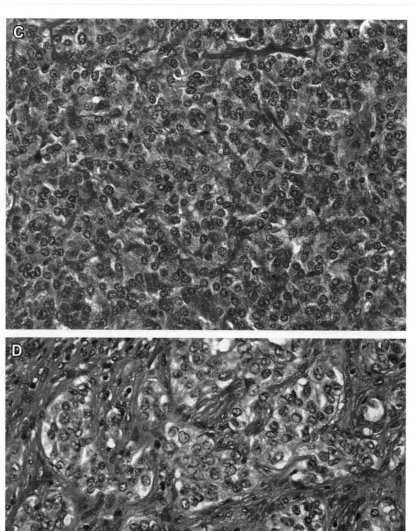

Fig. 18. (*C*) A peripancreatic pheochromocytoma demonstrating organoid architecture mimicking nested pattern of PanNET. (*D*) An unusual morphology of a ductal carcinoma of the pancreas demonstrating solid and nested pattern with low to moderate grade nuclear atypia.

admixed with an acinar cell carcinoma with a varying degree of NE differentiation evident by immunohistochemistry. The presence of more than 25% tumor cells with NE marker expression in an acinar cell carcinoma is considered a combined acinar cell carcinoma and high-grade NE carcinoma.[2] High-grade NE carcinoma is usually immunoreactive to pancytokeratin and chromogranin/synaptophysin although not in a diffusely intense pattern due to its poorly differentiated nature. Immunohistochemistry for trypsin and chymotrypsin should be performed to exclude acinar cell carcinoma. The Ki-67 proliferative index in a high-grade NE carcinoma is usually greater than 70% with a relatively homogenous expression throughout the tumor. Because the subtype

Fig. 19. Metastatic renal cell carcinoma to pancreas. (*A*) Renal cell carcinoma (two foci) metastatic to the pancreas with a heterogeneous gross appearance admixed with hemorrhage and bright yellow tumor parenchyma. (*B*) Renal cell carcinoma exhibits abundant vasculature and hemorrhage. (*C*) Nested tumor cells reveal atypical nuclei with nucleoli and clear cytoplasm.

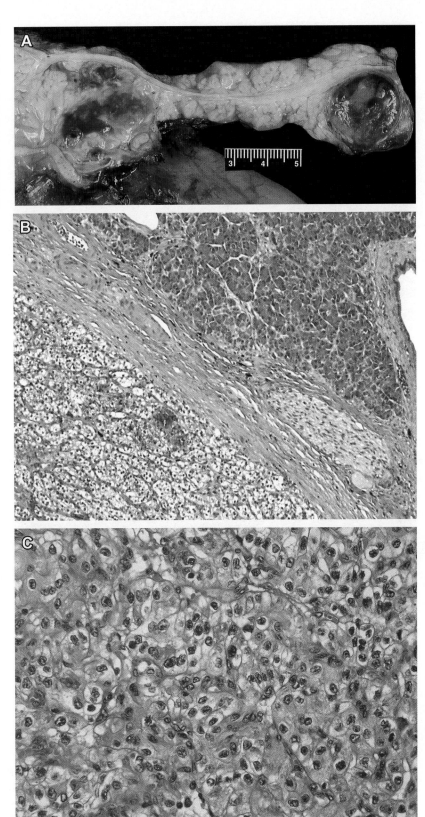

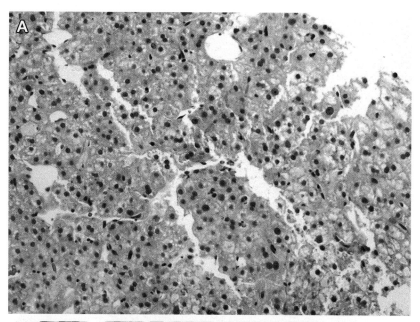

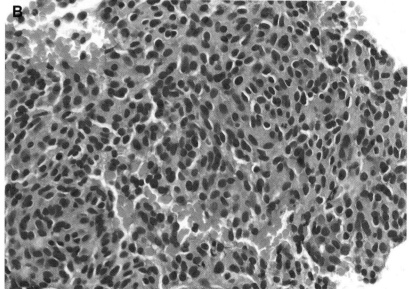

Fig. 20 part I. Differential diagnosis of Pan-NET in the liver (I). (*A*) Hepatocellular carcinoma with loosely cohesive architecture and abundant eosinophilic cytoplasm. (*B*) Metastatic atypical carcinoid tumor of lung with spindle cell morphology and rare identifiable mitosis.

of high-grade NE carcinoma is more common in the lung, a pulmonary metastasis to the liver and the pancreas should be considered in the differential diagnosis. The combined radiographic evidence of a lung mass and positive immunoreactivity for TTF1 supports a pulmonary origin although TTF1 can be positive in a pancreatic or gastrointestinal primary high-grade NE carcinoma, particularly the small cell variant.[18] Pitfalls in diagnosis of Pan-NET and common sources of diagnostic error are summarized in the Pitfalls box at the end of the article.

Fig. 20 part I. (C) Metastatic well-differentiated NET (carcinoid tumor) from small bowel showing combined nested and glandular architecture with peripheral serotonin containing granulated cells yielding the appearance of palisading. *(D)* Metastatic medullar thyroid carcinoma with spindled and a whorling morphologic pattern and rich vasculature.

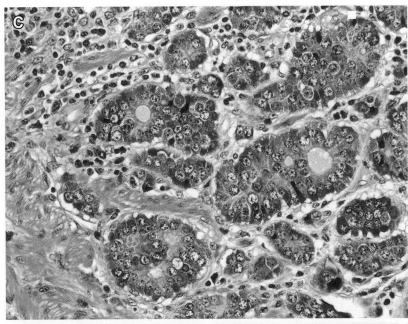

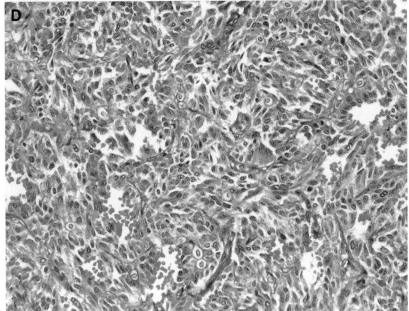

GRADING AND STAGING

In general, NETs are divided into well-differentiated and poorly differentiated categories. Differentiation refers to the extent to which the neoplastic cells resemble their non-neoplastic counterparts (eg, islet cells in cases of pancreatic origin). In NETs, well-differentiated examples exhibit characteristic pathologic features and contain NE secretory granules in the cytoplasm. This is reflected by diffuse and strong immunoreactivity for NE markers, such as chromogranin-A and synaptophysin.

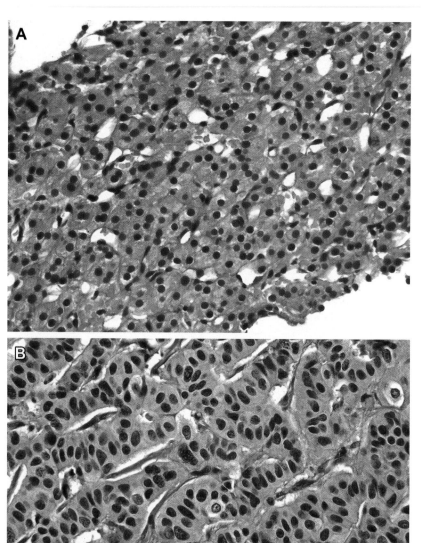

Fig. 20 *part II.* Differential diagnosis of Pan-NET in the liver (II). (*A*) Metastatic adrenal cortical carcinoma with an epithelioid morphology, eosinophilic cytoplasm, and rich vasculature. (*B*) Metastatic ductal carcinoma of the breast with an unusual nested and trabecular architecture and relatively low nuclear grade mimicking a well-differentiated NET.

Poorly differentiated NE carcinomas do not closely resemble any non-neoplastic epithelial cell counterparts and have high-grade cytologic features with only partial expression of NE markers on immunohistochemistry.

Grade, on the contrary, refers to the inherent malignant potential of the tumor. Low-grade NETs (no necrosis and less than two mitoses/50 HPF) are relatively indolent whereas high-grade NE carcinomas are extremely aggressive, and intermediate-grade examples (necrosis or 2 to 50 mitoses/50 HPF) have less predictable course. In general, well-differentiated NETs are either low grade or intermediate grade, and poorly

Fig. 20 part II. (*C*) Metastatic melanoma with nested architecture, plasmacytoid cytologic features, and marked nuclear atypia. (*D*) Primary angiomyolipoma of the liver with loosely cohesive epitheliod cells and abundant and condensed eosinophilic cytoplasm.

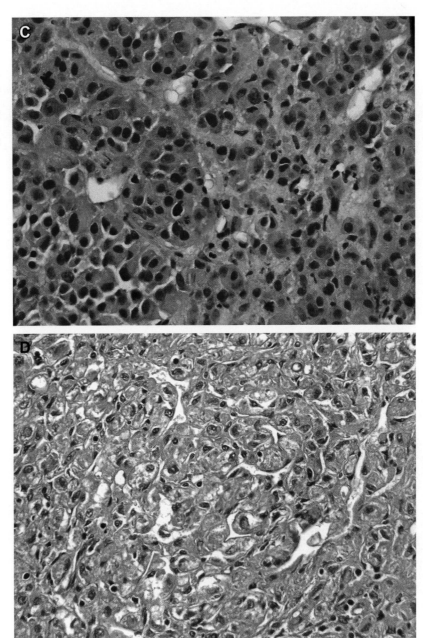

differentiated NETs are inevitably and uniformly high grade. The American Joint Committee on Cancer (AJCC) has recently published a TNM staging manual that includes NETs of all anatomic sites, which is somewhat different, particularly for the primary tumors of the pancreas, from the previously published European Neuroendocrine Tumor Society (ENETS) recommendations for TNM staging for gastrointestinal tract and the pancreatic NETs.[8,23,24] The staging criteria for both AJCC and ENETS, however, principally rely on tumor size and the extent of invasion into similar landmarks structures, which are used for the staging of non-NE carcinomas of the same sites. It is thus recommended that the extent of involvement of these structures be specifically

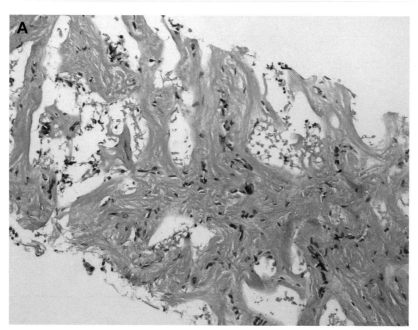

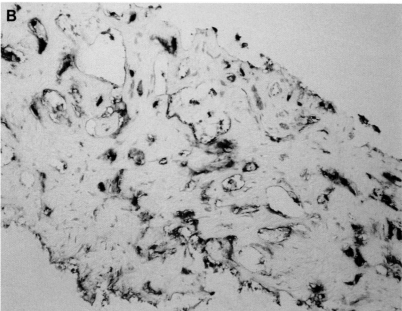

Fig. 21. Pan-NET with a pattern of a pseudodovascular lesion in liver biopsy. (*A*) Prominent vascular spaces with a few attached and crush tumor cells yielding an appearance of a benign hemangioma. (*B*) An immunostain for synaptophysin identifies the neoplastic cells.

indicated in the pathology reports, in addition to providing a TNM stage based on a system that is specifically referenced.[11]

Recently, a multidisciplinary consensus group comprised of NET experts in the field developed a minimum pathology data set of features to be included in pathology reports.[11] The College of American Pathologists has also developed similar tumor checklists for NETs that specify many of the same parameters.[10,19,20,22,24–28]

The pathologic classification of Pan-NET generally is comparable with that of NETs in the gastrointestinal tract with some notable differences and separate TNM staging systems. The issue of

Fig. *22.* Pan-NET with crush artifact in a small biopsy. (*A*) Crush artifact creates an impression of a high-grade NE carcinoma. (*B*) A Ki-67 immunostain confirms the low-grade nature of this well-differentiated Pan-NET with less than 2% nuclear immunoreactivity.

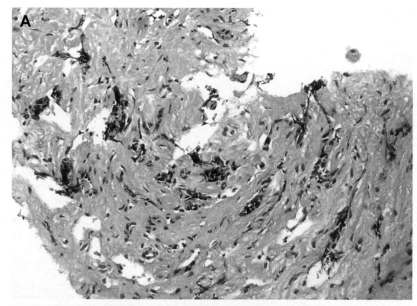

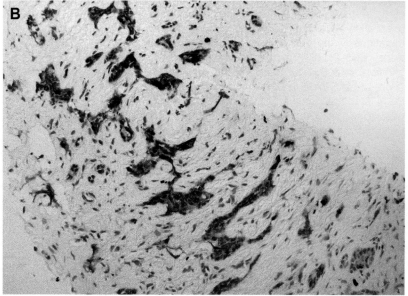

functionality of NETs also has an impact on the nomenclature for Pan-NETs because functioning Pan-NETs are defined based on the presence of clinical symptoms due to excess hormone secretion by the tumor. Terms reflecting the clinical syndromes (insulinoma, glucagonoma, VIPoma, gastrinoma, and so forth) may be applied to this group of NETs.[20]

MOLECULAR CHARACTERISTICS

Cytogenetic and molecular genetic studies have identified many chromosomal alterations in Pan-NETS but activation of oncogenes does not seem to play a major role in their development. Many of the genes targeted in the development of ductal adenocarcinoma of the pancreas, in particular, *KRAS2*, *TP53*, *p16/cdkn2A*, and *SMAD4*, are not mutated in most Pan-NETs.[25,29] Alternatively, biallelic inactivation of the *MEN1* gene, usually through a mutation in one allele coupled with loss of the remaining wild-type allele, occurs in 25% to 30% of Pan-NETs.[30,31] Also, even though *VHL* gene is usually not targeted in sporadic Pan-NETs,[24,32] Pan-NETs arising in patients with the vHL syndrome usually show biallelic inactivation of the *VHL* gene.[33]

Chromosomal gains and losses and expression analyses have revealed candidate loci for genes involved in the development of Pan-NETs.[34–36] A recent genomic sequencing project on nonfunctional Pan-NETs has identified that 44% of the tumors had somatic inactivating mutations in *MEN1,* which encodes menin, a component of a histone methyltransferase complex; and 43% had mutations in genes encoding either of the two subunits of a transcription/chromatin remodeling complex consisting of death-domain associated protein (DAXX) and -thalassemia/mental retardation syndrome X-linked (ATRX). Clinically, mutations in the *MEN1* and *DAXX/ATRX* genes were associated with better prognosis.[37] In addition, mutations in genes in the mammalian target of rapamycin (mTOR) pathway were found in 14% of the tumors. This observation could potentially be used to stratify patients for treatment with mTOR inhibitors.

PROGNOSIS

As is the case for other well-differentiated endocrine neoplasms, the natural history of Pan-NET is often unpredictable. Small Pan-NETs that do not exhibit adverse prognostic features (discussed later) can be cured by surgical resection. Many insulinomas fit this category, because they are generally less than 2 cm when detected. Most Pan-NETs other than insulinomas, however, are usually larger at the time of initial diagnosis, and the prognosis for this group is usually much less favorable. Approximately 50% to 80% of these neoplasms recur or metastasize, although sometimes such events may happen many years later.[3] Thus, studies with short follow-up often underestimate the proportion of Pan-NETs that ultimately behave in a malignant fashion. The 5-year survival after surgical resection for nonfunctional Pan-NETs is 65%, and the 10-year survival is 45%.[3] Pan-NETs are not sensitive to conventional chemotherapy, and cure is generally not possible after the development of metastases.

Although efforts to classify Pan-NETs into prognostically distinct subgroups have been of limited

Pitfalls
COMMON SOURCES OF DIAGNOSTIC ERROR

Failure to:

! Provide or recognize tumor differentiation and tumor grade (well vs poorly differentiated; low/intermediate grade vs high grade). These criteria are critical for determining therapeutic strategy.

! Recognize and accept atypical morphology in a well-differentiated Pan-NET and, therefore, misinterpret the appearance as indicative of a poorly differentiated ductal carcinoma or undifferentiated carcinoma. This results in inappropriate therapy.

! Consider a nonepithelial NE tumor (pheochromocytoma). This may result in significant clinical consequences (eg, hypertensive crisis).

! Provide an appropriate list of differential diagnoses during the case work-up.

! Adequately interpolate clinical information with the pathologic assessment.

! Assess or interpret tumor immunohistochemistry without adequate consideration of the entire morphologic picture.

success, many studies concur with respect to the criteria most predictive of recurrence or metastasis after surgical resection. The features that are well recognized as having prognostic significance in Pan-NETs include

1. Tumor size
2. Mitotic rate
3. Presence of necrosis
4. Extrapancreatic invasion
5. Vascular invasion
6. Nodal metastases
7. Distant metastases.

The grading of Pan-NETs based on the presence of either necrosis or a mitotic rate of greater than or equal to 2 per 50 HPFs stratifies the neoplasms into low-grade and intermediate-grade categories, which have highly significant differences in disease-free and disease-specific survival.[16] Increased Ki-67 labeling index has also been reportedly predictive of more aggressive behavior.[34,38]

REFERENCES

1. Nicholls AG. Simple adenoma of the pancreas arising from an island of langerhans. J Med Res 1902;8:385.

2. Hruban RH, Pitman MB, Klimstra D. Tumor of the Pancreas. AFIP atlas of tumor pathology, Series 4. 6th edition. Washington, DC: American Registry of Pathology; 2007.

3. Ferrone CR, Tang LH, Tomlinson J, et al. Determining prognosis in patients with pancreatic endocrine neoplasms: can the WHO classification system be simplified? J Clin Oncol 2007;25(35):5609–15.

4. Hussain S, Arwini A, Chetty R, et al. Oncocytic pancreatic endocrine neoplasms: a clinicopathologic and immunohistochemical analysis of 21 cases. Mod Pathol 2005;18:279A.

5. Hoang MP, Hruban RH, Albores-Saavedra J. Clear cell endocrine pancreatic tumor mimicking renal cell carcinoma: a distinctive neoplasm of von Hippel-Lindau disease. Am J Surg Pathol 2001;25(5):602–9.

6. Zee SY, Hochwald SN, Conlon KC, et al. Pleomorphic pancreatic endocrine neoplasms: a variant commonly confused with adenocarcinoma. Am J Surg Pathol 2005;29(9):1194–200.

7. Rindi G, de Herder WW, O'Toole D, et al. Consensus guidelines for the management of patients with digestive neuroendocrine tumors: why such guidelines and how we went about It. Neuroendocrinology 2006;84(3):155–7.

8. Kulke MH, Anthony LB, Bushnell DL, et al. NANETS treatment guidelines: well-differentiated neuroendocrine tumors of the stomach and pancreas. Pancreas 2010;39(6):735–52.

9. Scarpa A, Mantovani W, Capelli P, et al. Pancreatic endocrine tumors: improved TNM staging and histopathological grading permit a clinically efficient prognostic stratification of patients. Mod Pathol 2010;23(6):824–33.

10. Washington K, Tang LH, Berlin J, et al. Protocol for the Examination of Specimens from Patients with Carcinoma or Endocrine Pancreas. Arch Pathol Lab Med, in press.

11. Klimstra DS, Modlin IR, Adsay NV, et al. Pathology reporting of neuroendocrine tumors: application of the Delphic consensus process to the development of a minimum pathology data set. Am J Surg Pathol 2010;34(3):300–13.

12. Kwekkeboom DJ, Krenning EP, Scheidhauer K, et al. ENETS Consensus Guidelines for the Standards of Care in Neuroendocrine Tumors: somatostatin receptor imaging with (111)In-pentetreotide. Neuroendocrinology 2009;90(2):184–9.

13. Carrasquillo JA, Chen CC. Molecular imaging of neuroendocrine tumors. Semin Oncol 2010;37(6):662–79.

14. Hicks R. Use of molecular targeted agents for the diagnosis, staging and therapy of neuroendocrine malignancy. Cancer Imaging 2010;10(Spec no A):S83–91.

15. Klimstra DS. Nonductal neoplasms of the pancreas. Mod Pathol 2007;20(Suppl 1):S94–112.

16. Hochwald SN, Zee S, Conlon KC, et al. Prognostic factors in pancreatic endocrine neoplasms: an analysis of 136 cases with a proposal for low-grade and intermediate-grade groups. J Clin Oncol 2002; 20(11):2633–42.

17. Tang LH, Shia J, Vakiani E, et al. Transforming High Grade Neuroendocrine Neoplasms (NENs) of the Enteropancreatic System—a Unique Entity Distinct from De Novo High Grade Neuroendocrine Carcinomas (HGNCa) on Pathogenesis and Clinical Behavior. Mod Pathol 2008;21:137.

18. Shia J, Tang LH, Weiser MR, et al. Is nonsmall cell type high-grade neuroendocrine carcinoma of the tubular gastrointestinal tract a distinct disease entity? Am J Surg Pathol 2008;32(5):719–31.

19. Nassar H, Albores-Saavedra J, Klimstra DS. Highgrade neuroendocrine carcinoma of the ampulla of vater: a clinicopathologic and immunohistochemical analysis of 14 cases. Am J Surg Pathol 2005;29(5): 588–94.

20. Sun W, Sneige N, Staerkel G. Comparison of endoscopic ultrasound-guided and computed tomography-guided fine needle aspiration biopsy in the diagnosis of islet cell tumor of the pancreas [abstract]. Mod Pathol 2004;17:82A.

21. Norton JA, Shawker TH, Doppman JL, et al. Localization and surgical treatment of occult insulinomas. Ann Surg 1990;212(5):615–20.

22. Klimstra DS, Pitman MB, Hruban RH. An algorithmic approach to the diagnosis of pancreatic neoplasms. Arch Pathol Lab Med 2009;133(3):454–64.

23. American Joint Cancer Committee (AJCC) Cancer Staging Manual. 7th edition. New York (NY): Springer; 2010.

24. Rindi G, Kloppel G, Alhman H, et al. TNM staging of foregut (neuro)endocrine tumors: a consensus proposal including a grading system. Virchows Arch 2006;449(4):395–401.

25. Gortz B, Roth J, Krahenmann A, et al. Mutations and allelic deletions of the MEN1 gene are associated with a subset of sporadic endocrine pancreatic and neuroendocrine tumors and not restricted to foregut neoplasms. Am J Pathol 1999;154(2):429–36.

26. Washington MK, Tang LH, Berlin J, et al. Protocol for the examination of specimens from patients with neuroendocrine tumors (carcinoid tumors) of the small intestine and ampulla. Arch Pathol Lab Med 2010;134(2):181–6.

27. Washington MK, Tang LH, Berlin J, et al. Protocol for the examination of specimens from patients with neuroendocrine tumors (carcinoid tumors) of the stomach. Arch Pathol Lab Med 2010;134(2):187–91.

28. Washington MK, Tang LH, Berlin J, et al. Protocol for the examination of specimens from patients with neuroendocrine tumors (carcinoid tumors) of the appendix. Arch Pathol Lab Med 2010;134(2): 171–5.

29. Pellegata NS, Sessa F, Renault B, et al. K-ras and p53 gene mutations in pancreatic cancer: ductal and nonductal tumors progress through different genetic lesions. Cancer Res 1994;54(6):1556–60.

30. Corbo V, Dalai I, Scardoni M, et al. MEN1 in pancreatic endocrine tumors: analysis of gene and protein status in 169 sporadic neoplasms reveals alterations in the vast majority of cases. Endocr Relat Cancer 2010;17(3):771–83.

31. Capelli P, Martignoni G, Pedica F, et al. Endocrine neoplasms of the pancreas: pathologic and genetic features. Arch Pathol Lab Med 2009;133(3):350–64.

32. Moore PS, Missiaglia E, Antonello D, et al. Role of disease-causing genes in sporadic pancreatic endocrine tumors: MEN1 and VHL. Genes Chromosomes Cancer 2001;32(2):177–81.

33. Lubensky IA, Pack S, Ault D, et al. Multiple neuroendocrine tumors of the pancreas in von Hippel-Lindau disease patients: histopathological and molecular genetic analysis. Am J Pathol 1998; 153(1):223–31.

34. Chung DC, Brown SB, Graeme-Cook F, et al. Localization of putative tumor suppressor loci by genome-wide allelotyping in human pancreatic endocrine tumors. Cancer Res 1998;58(16):3706–11.

35. Floridia G, Grilli G, Salvatore M, et al. Chromosomal alterations detected by comparative genomic hybridization in nonfunctioning endocrine pancreatic tumors. Cancer Genet Cytogenet 2005;156(1): 23–30.

36. Hu W, Feng Z, Modica I, et al. Gene amplifications in well-differentiated pancreatic neuroendocrine tumors inactivate the p53 pathway. Genes Cancer 2010;1(4):360–8.

37. Jiao Y, Shi C, Edil BH, et al. DAXX/ATRX, MEN1 and mTOR pathway genes are frequently altered in pancreatic neuroendocrine tumors. Science 2011; 331(6021):1199–203.

38. Ekeblad S, Skogseid B, Dunder K, et al. Prognostic factors and survival in 324 patients with pancreatic endocrine tumor treated at a single institution. Clin Cancer Res 2008;14(23):7798–803.

PANCREATITIS, OTHER INFLAMMATORY LESIONS, AND PANCREATIC PSEUDOTUMORS

Alton B. Farris III, MD[a],*, Olca Basturk, MD[b], N. Volkan Adsay, MD[c]

KEYWORDS

- Pancreatitis • Diabetes • Pseudotumors • Pathology • Pancreas • Inflammatory lesions
- Autoimmune

ABSTRACT

The pancreas is versatile in the diversity of disorders that it can exhibit. In this article, characteristics of disorders such as chronic, autoimmune, eosinophilic, hereditary, and infectious pancreatitis are described. With regard to autoimmune pancreatitis, the role of clinical evaluation, histologic examination, and IgG4 immunohistochemistry is discussed. The role of pancreatitis in the pathogenesis of diabetes is also mentioned. Some implications of pancreatitis are highlighted, including the neoplastic predisposition caused by inflammatory lesions of the pancreas. The goal of this article is to convey an appreciation of these disorders because recognizing these disorders can benefit patients tremendously, as inflammatory lesions of the pancreas can be mass-forming, giving rise to pseudotumors, leading to surgical resection that may otherwise be unnecessary.

OVERVIEW: INFLAMMATORY LESIONS OF THE PANCREAS

The pancreas is a complex organ owing to the large number of neoplastic, inflammatory, and pseuodoneoplastic lesions that it may contain. Because of its important endocrine and exocrine functions and its central anatomic location, abnormalities in the pancreas can manifest in a dramatic fashion. This article focuses on inflammatory lesions of the pancreas as well as some benign pancreatic lesions that may be mistaken for neoplasia by clinicians, radiologists, and even pathologists. The article attempts to aid the pathologist in confronting the differential diagnosis of these important entities.

INFLAMMATORY LESIONS OF THE PANCREAS

ACUTE PANCREATITIS

Acute pancreatitis (**Fig. 1**) is characterized clinically by upper abdominal pain, epigastric pain, and pancreatic enzyme (lipase or amylase [hyperamylasemia]) elevation, detectable in either the blood or urine. Other signs and symptoms may be present including nausea, vomiting, and fever. Abnormal laboratory values that may also be present include a transient hyperglycemia, hypertriglyceridemia, and hypocalcemia.[1,2] Criteria used for the prediction of pancreatitis severity include the Atlanta classification,[3] Ranson's

Disclosures: None.
[a] Department of Pathology and Laboratory Medicine, Emory University Hospital, Emory University, 1364 Clifton Road Northeast, Room H-188, Atlanta, GA 30322, USA
[b] Department of Pathology, Memorial Sloan-Kettering Cancer Center, 1275 York Avenue, New York, NY 10065, USA
[c] Department of Pathology and Laboratory Medicine, Emory University, 1364 Clifton Road NE, Room H-180B, Atlanta, GA 30322, USA
* Corresponding author.
E-mail address: abfarri@emory.edu

Surgical Pathology 4 (2011) 625–650
doi:10.1016/j.path.2011.03.004

surgpath.theclinics.com

Key Points
PANCREATITIS

- Acute and chronic pancreatitis have commonalities and likely represent a continuum between each other.

- Alcohol use is a common contributor to both acute and chronic pancreatitis.

- Autoimmune pancreatitis has been the focus of much interest recently. A diagnostic feature of most autoimmune pancreatitis cases is an increased number of immunoglobulin (Ig) G4+ plasma cells amidst a prominent lymphoplasmacytic infiltrate.

- The family of pancreatic "pseudotumors," by a loosely defined conception of that term, includes a variety of lesions that must be clearly delineated. Knowledge of these entities, as mentioned in the differential diagnosis, will help in making an accurate diagnosis.

- Pancreatitis may lead to an increased risk for the development of pancreatic carcinoma.

Differential Diagnosis
PANCREATITIS, INFLAMMATORY LESIONS, AND PSEUDOTUMORS

- The differential diagnosis of inflammatory lesions and pseudotumors of the pancreas is broad, including both benign and malignant lesions.

- Autoimmune pancreatitis (AIP) is an important type of pancreatitis that must be recognized. Recently, an expert panel has suggested the use of the terms *Type 1 AIP* for cases that used to be called lymphoplasmacytic sclerosing pancreatitis (LPSP) (AIP without granulocytic epithelial lesions [GELs]) and *Type 2 AIP* for cases that used to be called idiopathic ductocentric pancreatitis (IDCP) (AIP with GELs).

- "Pseudotumors" should be kept in the differential diagnosis when a pancreatic mass is encountered. Loosely, these include pseudocysts, retention cysts, lymphoepithelial cysts, ampullary adenoma, splenic heterotopia, hamartoma, and lipomatous pseudohypertrophy. Paraduodenal ("groove") pancreatitis may lead to cystic change and pseudotumor formation.

- The differential diagnostic considerations for cystic pancreatic lesions are important to recall when assessing cystic pancreatic lesions. The list of possibilities includes both inflammatory lesions and epithelial "neoplasms."

criteria,[4] and the Acute Physiology and Chronic Health Evaluation (APACHE) grading system.[1,2,4–6]

Acute pancreatitis has a number of etiologic associations, some of which may overlap with chronic pancreatitis. Choledocholithiasis is the most common cause of acute pancreatitis, in which women are affected more than men and the peak affected age is between 50 and 60 years. Alcohol is the second most common cause of pancreatitis, affecting men more than women.[1,2,7] Together, cholelithiasis and alcohol consumption account for 70% to 80% of acute pancreatitis cases.[1,8,9] Other causes may be associated with pancreatitis, including hyperlipidemia, certain drugs (particularly as an effect of treatment for the acquired immune deficiency syndrome [AIDS]), certain infectious agents (see later in this article), and autoimmune disease (eg, systemic lupus erythematosis [SLE]).[1,8] Anatomic abnormalities such as pancreas divisum may predispose patients to pancreatitis, particularly recurrent pancreatitis.[10] About 10% of cases are idiopathic.[8]

Acute pancreatitis is classified as either acute interstitial or acute hemorrhagic types. Acute hemorrhagic pancreatitis consists of necrotizing pancreatitis owing to disruption of the pancreatic microcirculation, typically leading to severe systemic complications, often requiring surgical intervention. Pancreatic and peripancreatic tissue hemorrhagic disruption may lead to accumulation of blood in the retroperitoneal space in the periumbilical of flank area, imparting a bluish discoloration known as the Gray-Turner or Cullen sign. Acute interstitial pancreatitis consists of acute pancreatic inflammation with or without peripancreatic inflammation and without disruption of the pancreatic microvasculature.[1,2]

Grossly, the pancreas is swollen and indurated in acute pancreatitis, and pancreatic lobules appear separated because interstitial spaces contain edema. There may be purulent material, fat necrosis appreciable as a white discoloration, and hemorrhage. Frank necrosis characterized by red to red-black discoloration may alternate with areas of more normal-appearing pancreatic tissue.[8]

Microscopic examination of biopsy material from cases of acute pancreatitis is not usually performed because the diagnosis of acute pancreatitis is usually made clinically. In acute interstitial pancreatitis, on microscopic examination, necrosis may be focal or diffuse. There is typically an acute inflammatory cell infiltrate admixed with

Fig. 1. Acute pancreatitis. (*A*) Acute hemorrhagic pancreatitis with necrosis of the pancreatic parenchyma and admixed hemorrhage (H&E, original magnification x5). (*B*) Higher power of the hemorrhagic necrosis showing areas of calcification (*arrow*) (H&E, original magnification x10).

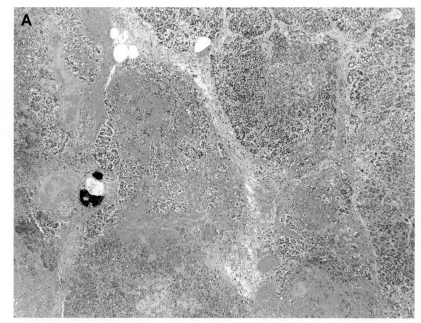

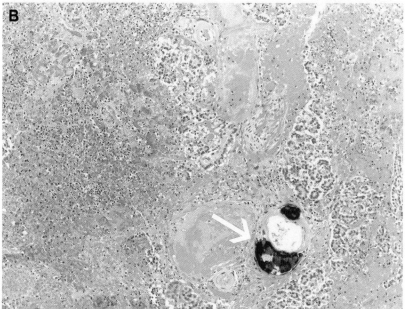

edema and fibrinous exudates. Pancreatic ducts may be dilated and may contain hyperplasia and/or mucinous and/or squamous metaplasia. Vascular thrombosis and necrotizing arteritis are not typically seen.[8] In acute hemorrhagic pancreatitis, patchy necrosis is present in all pancreatic components, including the vascular structures, ducts, acini, islets of Langerhans, nerves, and adipose tissue, typically in a periductal or perilobular distribution with a sparing of portions of the pancreas. Minimal inflammation is present early in the process; later, the quantity of inflammation increases, with a predominance of acute inflammatory cells. Vascular thrombosis may also be seen.[8] Fat necrosis may be seen in association with acute pancreatitis, and there may also be organization of pancreatic abscesses and pseudocyst formation.[8]

Acute pancreatitis is typically treated with supportive care, including fluid replacement, pain relief (typically meperidine), and avoidance of oral alimentation to reduce pancreatic secretion.[7,9] Antibiotic therapy may be helpful in some cases.[11]

CHRONIC PANCREATITIS

Chronic pancreatitis (**Fig. 2**) is a fibroinflammatory disorder of the pancreas resulting in permanent functional impairment with the clinical triad of steatorrhea, diabetes, and pancreatic calcification on radiographic studies.[12,13] Alcohol ingestion is the most common cause of chronic pancreatitis, comprising about 70% of cases; however, only about 10% of alcohol abusers develop chronic pancreatitis. Alcohol-related chronic pancreatitis shows a male predilection and predominance in the fourth to sixth decade age group.[14–18] Cigarette smoking also contributes to the development

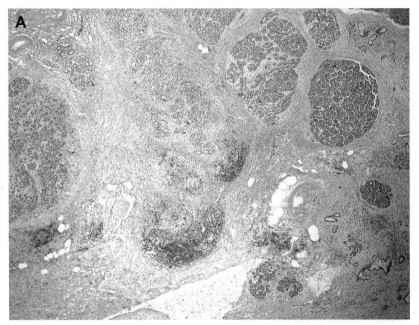

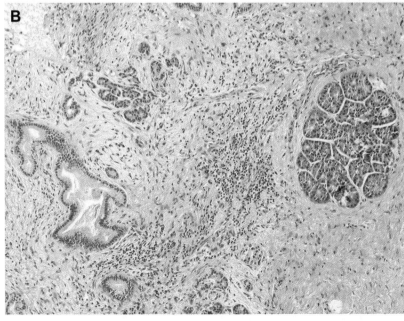

Fig. 2. Chronic pancreatitis. (*A*) Low power of a case of chronic pancreatitis showing prominent fibrosis and admixed chronic inflammatory cells and parenchymal atrophy (H&E, original magnification x2). (*B*) Higher power of chronic pancreatitis showing fibrosis, chronic inflammation, and acinar atrophy (H&E, original magnification x10).

of chronic pancreatitis.[18,19] The genetic disorder cystic fibrosis leads to an increased risk for the development of chronic pancreatitis, together with pancreatic insufficiency.[20] Ultimately, about 10% to 25% of cases have an idiopathic etiology; however, some of the cases that were previously referred to as "idiopathic" are now thought to represent cases of autoimmune pancreatitis.[20]

Several classification systems have been developed to classify chronic pancreatitis, including the Marseille classification (1963), the revised Marseille classification (1983), the Marseille-Rome classification (1988), the Cambridge classification (1997), the Zurich classification (1997), and the Japan Pancreas Society classification (1997). The Marseille and revised Marseille classifications are considered to be outdated. The Zurich Classification System has categories for alcohol and nonalcohol-related chronic pancreatitis, and the Japan Society Classification system places more emphasis on a variety of diagnostic criteria without emphasis on etiology. Both of these systems have categories for both "definite" and "probable" chronic pancreatitis. Overall, there is still a lack of good criteria for chronic pancreatitis.[12,13]

Clinically, patients with chronic pancreatitis have abdominal pain, weight loss, and malabsorption, often with steatorrhea. There may be pancreatic masses, pseudocysts or abscesses, pleural effusions, gastrointestinal bleeding, and peptic ulceration. Pancreatic endocrine insufficiency may develop, including diabetes.[21] CA19-9 serum levels may be elevated and pleural effusions may have elevated amylase levels.[22,23] Calcifications may be detected radiographically in cases of chronic pancreatitis.[24] Some cases of chronic pancreatitis may be associated with hypercalcemic syndromes (ie, hyperparathyroidism); and in these cases, the pathologic changes in the pancreas may be indistinguishable from alcoholic chronic pancreatitis.[14,20,25,26]

Upon gross examination, there is focal, segmental, or diffuse enlargement; induration; and/or fibrosis of the pancreas. There may be irregular cystic dilatation of the pancreatic ducts, which may contain calcified proteins (calculi). Atrophy may be so extensive that the pancreas may become shrunken and hardened. Pseudocyst formation with necrotic/hemorrhagic debris may be present.[20]

Microscopically, there are variable degrees of atrophy in chronic pancreatitis with loss of acinar and ductal tissue, chronic inflammation, and fibrosis with a preservation of the lobular architecture of the pancreatic gland. Chronic pancreatitis may sometimes be confused with pancreatic ductal adenocarcinoma; however, the preserved lobular architecture of chronic pancreatitis helps a pathologist make a proper benign diagnosis. Ductal dilatation and ectasia, cyst formation, calculi, and inspissated secretions may be present.[20,27] Calculi are usually composed of calcium carbonate (about 80% of the time) and range in size from less than 1 mm to more than 1 cm in diameter.[14] Ductal hyperplasia (papillary or pseudopapillary), metaplasia (eg, squamous, mucous cell, or pyloric gland), or atrophy may be present. In pancreatitis from chronic obstruction (also known as "chronic obstructive pancreatitis") in particular, ductal hyperplasia may be observed, together with ductal dilatation distal to the obstruction, fibrosis, and acinar atrophy. Large ducts may have saccular dilatations. Mucous cell metaplasia in some cases identical to what would be called pancreatic intraepithelial neoplasia (PanIN), type 1B, may be present. Reactive ductal epithelial changes may be identified with enlarged nuclei and irregular nuclear size, shape, and chromatin distribution; however, the changes seen in ductal adenocarcinoma are lacking, such as increased nuclear to cytoplasmic ratio, nuclear pleomorphism, crowding, stratification, increased mitotic rate, loss of lobular architecture, cribriforming, and desmoplasia.[20,27] However, these differences can be particularly difficult to distinguish on frozen sections.[28,29]

Chronic inflammation is often present, and perineural and intraneural inflammation can be seen, sometimes with hyperplasia of the nerves. The islets of Langerhans may be relatively preserved; however, hyperplasia or loss may be seen, with loss usually preferentially occurring in the insulin-producing cells.[20,27,30] Pancreatic polypeptide and glucagon-producing cells are usually increased without an appreciable change in the somatostatin-producing cells. Islet aggregation, which is characterized by a clustering of non-neoplastic islets, may be seen in chronic pancreatitis; such aggregates can be seen in the peripancreatic adipose tissue, leading to them being mistaken for an infiltrative epithelial process (ie, exocrine or endocrine carcinoma). Islet aggregation may have a misshapen, pseudoinfiltrative pattern, sometimes resulting from the presence of collagenized stroma around their periphery; and they may be present in close apposition to nerves, leading to a mimic of perineural "invasion," or adjacent to small ducts, resembling those seen in nesidioblastosis.[31–33] The tissue injury in acute pancreatitis usually recovers without residual signs of morphologic abnormality; however, the morphologic signs of injury usually persist after chronic pancreatitis.[20,27,34]

Chronic Tropical Pancreatitis

Chronic tropical pancreatitis typically presents in younger individuals and is not related to alcohol use. It usually presents in India, southern Asia, central Africa, and Brazil. This disorder has a diabetic phase that is commonly called fibrocalculous pancreatic diabetes. Chronic tropical pancreatitis typically consists of a triad of diabetes, abdominal pain, and steatorrhea. Although the precise etiology is unclear, factors thought to play a role in chronic tropical pancreatitis include dietary cyanogen toxicity, malnutrition, antioxidant deficiency, and a genetic predisposition (including mutations in the pancreatic secretory trypsin inhibitor gene and other genes). There may be large intraductal calculi. There is an increased preponderance to develop pancreatic cancer. Patients must be treated to control the concurrent diabetes that often develops because complications of diabetes are the leading cause of mortality and morbidity (eg, diabetic nephropathy).[35–41]

Grossly, the pancreas is often shrunken, firm, and nodular. The surface is often gritty, likely because of the presence of numerous pancreatic calculi of different sizes and shapes located diffusely throughout dilated pancreatic ducts. Pancreatic ducts often contain denuded epithelium and/or squamous metaplasia, and there is often a lymphoplasmacytic infiltrate, commonly periductal. There may be acinar cell atrophy and interlobular or diffuse fibrosis. Islets are often atrophic, surrounded by dense fibrosis.[35–41]

INFECTIOUS PANCREATITIS

Certain infectious agents can cause pancreatitis, particularly acute pancreatitis.[1,27,42] Infectious pancreatitis should particularly be suspected in immunocompromised patients, such as patients who have had an organ transplant or patients with acquired immunodeficiency syndrome (AIDS) because their acute pancreatitis incidence is higher than in healthy individuals.[43–46] Particular viral pathogens are of special consideration in the pancreas, including mumps,[47] coxsackievirus,[48,49] Epstein-Barr virus (EBV), rubella, cytomegalovirus (CMV), herpes simplex virus, hepatitis A and B, and HIV. The following bacteria are noteworthy for their involvement of the pancreas: *Mycobacterium tuberculosis,*[50] *Mycobacterium avium* complex, *Salmonella typhi, Campylobacter jejuni, Mycoplasma pneumoniae, Yersinia enterocolitica, Actinomyces,* and *Nocardia.* Fungal organisms, such as *Coccidioides immitis, Histoplasma capsulatum, Aspergillus, Cryptococcus neoformans, Pneumocystis jiroveci* (previously known as *carinii*), and *Paracoccidioides brasiliensis,* can involve the pancreas.[51] Parasites may also be seen in the pancreas, such as *Echinococcus granulosus, Ascaris lumbricoides,*[52] *Clonorchis sinensis,*[53–56] and *Strongyloides stercoralis.*[57,58] *Clonorchis* may be associated with extrahepatic cholangiocarcinoma.[53]

Patients with AIDS may be particularly susceptible to disseminated CMV infections[44] and also may characteristically have *Toxoplasma gondii,*[59] *Cryptococcus,*[60] *Cryptosporidium, M avium* complex, and *M tuberculosis.*[43–46] See **Table 1** for a summary of causes typically associated with pancreatitis.

Microscopically, certain infectious causes of pancreatitis have noteworthy findings. CMV inclusions may be appreciated in mesenchymal cells most often but may also be seen in epithelial cells

---

Table 1
Causes typically associated with acute pancreatitis, chronic pancreatitis, and both acute and chronic pancreatitis[a]

Acute and Chronic Pancreatitis	Acute Pancreatitis	Chronic Pancreatitis
• Ethanol (alcohol)-related	• Choledocholithiasis	• Cystic fibrosis
• Anatomic abnormalities (eg, paraduodenal pancreatitis, pancreas divisum, choledochal cysts)	• Drug-associated (eg, drugs used for AIDS treatment)	• Long-term insulin-dependent diabetes mellitus
• Metabolic (hypercalcemia, hyperlipidemia)	• Infectious 　○ Viral (eg, HIV) 　○ Parasites (eg, ascariasis) 　○ Bacteria (eg, *Mycoplasma*)	• Hemochromatosis • Tropical
• Autoimmune (eg, systemic lupus erythematosus)		• Familial/hereditary
• Obstruction		• Idiopathic
• Trauma		

[a] The most common causes of acute and chronic pancreatitis are listed, along with disorders commonly associated with both acute and chronic pancreatitis; however, it can be recognized that there is significant overlap.

(ie, acinar cells). Mycobacterial infection may lead to necrotizing or non-necrotizing granulomatous inflammation. *A lumbricoides* is the most common cause of parasitic pancreatitis and typically involves the pancreas through the pancreatic ductal system, leading to abscess formation, necrosis, fibrosis, granulomatous inflammation, and deposition of eggs and larvae.[52] Findings of specific organisms may not always be appreciable microscopically, and cultures may be required to diagnose infectious pancreatitis.[27]

Differential diagnostic considerations for infectious pancreatitis include rheumatoid arthritis, Crohn disease, and sarcoidosis.[61–64] Rheumatoid arthritis can lead to the presence of rheumatoid nodules in the pancreas.[51]

AUTOIMMUNE PANCREATITIS

Autoimmune pancreatitis (AIP) is a pancreatobiliary-centric inflammatory disease, **(Table 2)**, which is frequently mass forming, constituting one-quarter of Whipple resections performed for benign conditions in North America.[65–68] The first descriptions of what has become known as AIP originally appeared in the 1950s, notably among patients with ulcerative colitis and pancreatitis,[69] and in the 1960s in patients with sclerosing pancreatitis and hypergammaglobulinemia.[70,71] AIP has been of particular interest to the pathology community in recent years,[65–68] with the term "autoimmune pancreatitis" being coined in the 1990s.[72]

IgG4-associated Autoimmune Pancreatitis

IgG4-associated autoimmune pancreatitis (**Fig. 3**) is an important category of autoimmune pancreatitis that has gained interest recently because it probably constitutes most AIP cases. Other terms used for this disorder in the literature include lymphoplasmacytic sclerosing pancreatitis (LPSP) with cholangitis, chronic sclerosing pancreatitis, and nonalcoholic duct destructive chronic pancreatitis.[20] Recently, an expert panel has suggested "Type 1" AIP terminology (AIP without granulocytic epithelial lesions [see later in this article]).[73] IgG4-associated autoimmune pancreatitis is often a multicentric disease as evidenced by the presence of extra-pancreatic manifestations in approximately one-third of cases, among which lesions of the biliary system and liver are quite noteworthy.[65,68] The disease can involve the bile ducts (sclerosing cholangitis),[74] gallbladder (lymphoplasmacytic sclerosing cholecystitis),[75] kidney (interstitial nephritis and pseudotumors),[76] the salivary glands in a disorder previously commonly referred to as a Kuttner tumor,[77] and the lungs (forming inflammatory masses).[65,66,78,79] Such multiorgan involvement may be part of a systemic IgG4-related disease, which has been termed

---

Table 2
Autoimmune pancreatitis: primary distinguishing features of major subtypes

Term	Type 1 AIP (LPSP, AIP without GELs)	Type 2 AIP (IDCP, AIP with GELs)
Clinicopathology[a]	• Somewhat older patients • Men more than women (about 3:1) • Systemic manifestations: Interstitial nephritis, salivary gland lesions, slerosing cholangitis, Sjögren-like syndrome	• Younger patients [mid 40s] • Equal number of men and women • Inflammatory bowel disease, possibly
Histology[a]	• Lymphoplasmacytic • Fibroinflammatory • Obliterative phlebitis and arterial involvement • May extend to peripancreatic tissues	• Lymphoplasmacytic with GELs • Fibroinflammatory but perhaps less prominently than Type 1 • Typically no obliterative phlebitis or arterial involvement • Typically limited to pancreas and not peripancreatic tissues
IgG4 + staining	• Abundant (>10 cells/high-power field)	• Few to none

Abbreviations: AIP, Autoimmune pancreatitis; GELs, granulocytic epithelial lesions; IDCP, idiopathic duct centric pancreatitis; LPSP, lymphoplasmacytic sclerosing pancreatitis.
  [a] Features are somewhat mixed, and the association with a particular subtype is still a matter of debate in some instances.

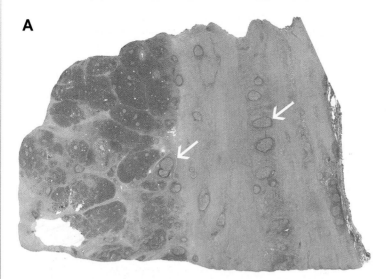

Fig. 3. Autoimmune pancreatitis. (A) Low power of an autoimmune pancreatitis case showing lymphoid nodules (*arrows*). (B) Low to medium power of an autoimmune pancreatitis case showing fibrosis, acinar atrophy, chronic inflammation, and periductal fibrosis (*arrow*). (C) Higher power showing periductal fibrosis. (All H&E.)

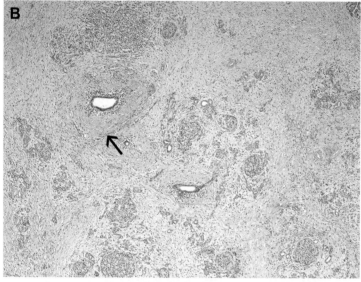

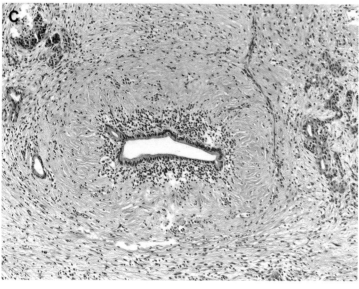

Fig. 3. (*D*) Higher power showing perineural inflammation (H&E). (*E*) Higher power showing lymphoplasmacytic infiltrate amidst storiform fibrosis (H&E). (*F*) IgG4 immunohistochemical stain at higher power, showing a number of IgG4+ plasma cells.

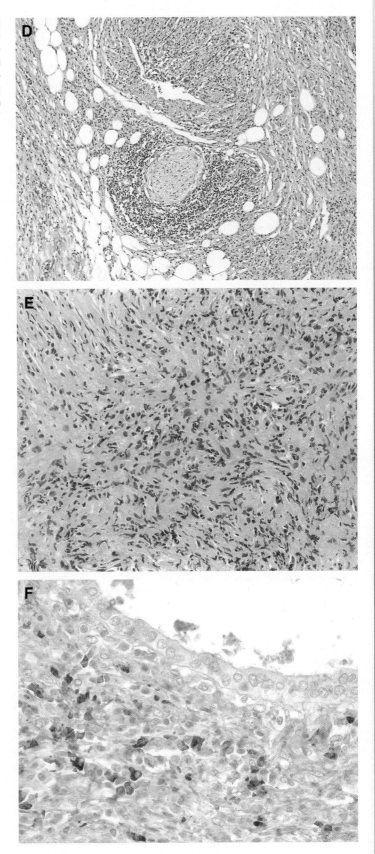

"IgG4-associated immune complex multiorgan autoimmune disease" (IMAD).[76]

Patients often present with vague abdominal pain; obstructive jaundice, when the disorder affects the bile ducts (75% to 80% of patients); and occasionally with other autoimmune diseases (in about 20% of patients and including such disorders as idiopathic retroperitoneal fibrosis, Sjögren's syndrome, ulcerative colitis, and lymphocytic thyroiditis). Later, middle age and elderly individuals are affected disproportionately.[66] Some patients with AIP may have diabetes.[80] Elevated levels of serum IgG4 can often be useful in recognizing the disease, and suspecting IgG4-associated disease is important because it is often responsive to steroid therapy.[81] The diagnosis can often be made before pancreatectomy using a combination of clinical findings, the presence of elevated IgG4 levels, radiologic features, response to steroids, and endoscopic ultrasound-guided fine-needle aspiration biopsy findings, potentially avoiding surgery in selected patients.[66,67] The presence of autoantibodies may be detected in the clinical laboratory, such as antinuclear antibodies (ANA), anti–smooth muscle antibodies, anticarbonic anhydrase II antibodies, and antilactoferrin antibodies.[82–84] Radiologic (eg, computed tomography, magnetic resonance imaging, or ultrasonography) studies often show a diffuse focal or segmental enlargement (mass formation) or hypoechoic enlargement of the pancreas (referred to as the "sausage sign") and may be useful in demonstrating a stenosis of bile/pancreatic ducts.[20,66,67] Endoscopic retrograde cholangiopancreatography (ERCP) can be used to recognize the disorder, often showing a diffusely irregular main pancreatic duct and strictures of the common bile duct.[66,67]

Grossly, the pancreas is most often noticeably abnormal in the head of the pancreas, where it is yellowish-white to gray, indurated, variably enlarged, and shows a loss of the normal lobular architecture. Bile duct/main pancreatic duct obstruction or stenosis may be observed, particularly in the distal portions, even extending to the papilla. Involvement in the tail, body, or diffusely throughout the pancreas is seen in a minority of cases. Pseudocysts are not usually seen, and calculi are uncommonly seen, typically only in advanced cases.[20,65,66]

Histologic findings in AIP are characterized by dense lymphoplasmacytic pancreatic parenchymal infiltrates with secondary fibrosis and acinar atrophy. Inflammation and injury may be spotty in an involved pancreas, showing prominently involved areas alternating with relatively uninvolved areas; and ducts are typically involved first followed by acinar involvement and sclerosis. The fibroinflammatory process involves the head of the pancreas in about 80% of cases; however, it can extend up the bile duct, leading to thickening of the bile duct and gallbladder walls and inflammation of the hilar tissues of the liver. Features of AIP include obliterative phlebitis and periductal inflammation forming a collar around small, medium-sized, and large interlobular ducts, with the smaller ducts being affected mostly in advanced cases. Perineural inflammation is also a useful feature in suggesting the diagnosis of AIP. Also, clues to the diagnosis of AIP are periductal granulomas and pseudotumors. Storiform fibrosis may be admixed with myofibroblast-type cells, leading to changes reminiscent of inflammatory pseudotumors.[20,65,66] Some studies have categorized cases of AIP into ductocentric (termed, "AIP-D"), characterized by fibroinflammatory processes primarily in the periductal region with or without lobular involvement, and lobulocentric ("AIP-L"), distinguished by having an almost exclusively lobular lymphoplasmacytic infiltrate with a paucity of periductal inflammation. In a study by Deshpande and colleagues,[65] the AIP-L group tended to have a higher proportion of male patients, more granulocytic epithelial lesions, less fibroblastic proliferation, and less IgG4.

Frank pseudotumor formation may occur, as evidenced in notable reports, and cases may be associated with idiopathic retroperitoneal fibrosis.[85–88] The pseudotumor formation may extend up the bile duct to involve the liver hilus, and there may be an overlap with cases previously referred to as primary sclerosing cholangitits.[74,89] Lymph nodes surrounding the pancreas and bile duct are commonly enlarged, showing follicular hyperplasia. Of note, typical stigmata of alcoholic pancreatitis are absent.[20,65,66]

The lymphoplasmacytic inflammation is characteristically composed of IgG4-positive plasma cells, and in addition, there may be admixed macrophages, neutrophils, and eosinophils. Vasculitis may involve small veins, and less commonly, arteries, sometimes leading to an obliterative arteritis. Lymphocytes are predominately CD4-positive and CD8-positive T cells with fewer B cells, and sometimes small follicles of B cells can be appreciated.[20,65,66] The number of IgG4-positive cells has varied according to different studies. Recent studies have suggested more than 10 IgG4-positive cells per high power field,[90] although others suggest a cutoff of greater than 20 IgG4 positive plasma cells gives a higher specificity.[91] In addition, using IgG4-positive cells as a surrogate marker of systemic disease has been suggested in different studies, some of which are depicted in **Table 3**.

Granulocytic Epithelial Lesion–forming (Idiopathic Ductcentric) Pancreatitis

A category of AIP in which the inflammatory infiltrate contains a pronounced component of neutrophils, which has been termed as a granulocytic epithelial lesion (GEL)-forming form of AIP (**Fig. 4**). Recently, an expert panel has recommended "Type 2" AIP (AIP with granulocytic epithelial lesions [see later in this article]).[73] GEL-forming AIP appears to occur in a younger subset of patients in their mid 40s and seems to affect equal numbers of men and women, unlike the other form of IgG4-associated AIP, which affects men more than women by a ratio of approximately 3:1. Cases with neutrophilic infiltrates also tend to be seen in younger individuals with inflammatory bowel disease as opposed to cases associated with Sjögren's syndrome, which affects older male patients preferentially and is not associated with pancreatic neutrophilic infiltrates.[20,92,93]

Histologically, the GEL-forming lesions are characterized by ductal epithelial detachment and injury secondary to invasion of the epithelium by neutrophils and sometimes eosinophils. Neutrophils and eosinophils may cluster underneath the epithelium, sometimes extending into small intralobular acini and ducts. Although the injury tends to be severe, it has been suggested that ductal scarring and complete obliteration are not common end points.[20,93]

Diagnosis of Autoimmune Pancreatitis Through Biopsy and Other Criteria

Since shortly after autoimmune pancreatitis gained attention as an entity, there has been interest in diagnosing autoimmune pancreatitis on the basis of biopsy material. The features typically associated with autoimmune pancreatitis can be appreciated on biopsies, notably the following: obliterative venulitis, granulocytic epithelial lesions, and periductal lymphocytic inflammation. Studies have investigated the use of IgG4 immunohistochemistry as an ancillary test to make the diagnosis of IgG4-associated autoimmune

Table 3
Autoimmune pancreatitis (AIP) and IgG4-mediated autoimmune disease diagnostic criteria using IgG4 immunohistochemistry in the pancreas and selected extrapancreatic organs

Specimen	Disease	Measure	References
Pancreas	AIP	≥5 IgG4+ plasma cell per 20x with all lobulocentric AIP >50 IgG4+ plasma cells/40x	65
	AIP	>20 IgG4+ plasma cells/HPF	98
	AIP	>10 IgG4+ plasma cells/HPF	95
	AIP	>10 IgG4+ plasma cells/HPF	90
Ampulla	AIP (surrogate marker)	IgG4+/IgG+ plasma cells = 0.10	99
Gallbladder	AIP (surrogate marker)	>10 IgG4+ plasma cells/HPF	75
Gallbladder	AIP (surrogate marker)	IgG4+/IgG+ plasma cells = 0.47	75
Liver	IgG4-associated cholangitis	>10 IgG4+ plasma cells/HPF in 6 of the IgG4-associated cholangitis cases	74
Salivary gland	Chronic sclerosing sialadenitis	Mean of 229 IgG4+ plasma cells/HPF and an overall IgG4/IgG ratio of 0.86	77
Kidney	IgG4 immune-complex tubulointerstitial nephritis pseudotumors	Numerous IgG4+ plasma cells in the infiltrate (immunohistochemistry or immunofluorescence)	76
Lung	AIP (surrogate marker)	All AIP cases stained had >10 IgG4+ plasma cells/HPF	78

Abbreviations: HPF, high-power field; Ig, immunoglobulin.

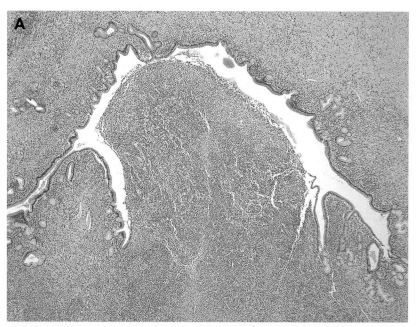

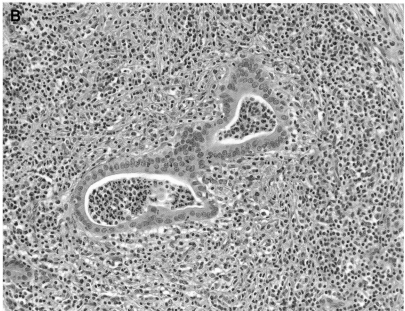

Fig. 4. Granulocytic epithelial lesion (GEL)-forming (idiopathic duct-centric) pancreatitis. (*A*) Medium power of a duct affected by a dense infiltrate of granulocytes, showing ductal epithelial destruction and inflammation. (*B*) Higher power of a duct containing luminal granulocytes, in a granulocytic epithelial lesion-forming pancreatitis case.

pancreatitis, but recommendations vary on the density of plasma cells that are needed to diagnose autoimmune pancreatitis, as shown in **Table 3**.[20,65,94–98] Studies have also recommended that a ratio of IgG4+ plasma cells to IgG+ plasma cells (obtained by counting the number of cells on both IgG4-stained and IgG-stained tissue sections) is more useful diagnostically, because in a sense this measures the percentage of IgG produced by plasma cells that is composed of IgG4. For the diagnosis of autoimmune pancreatitis, it has been proposed that this IgG4:IgG ratio can be useful as a surrogate marker of disease in the pancreas in ampullary biopsies[99] and cholecystectomy specimens (**Table 3**).[75] Multiple criteria sets have been developed to assist in the diagnosis of autoimmune pancreatitis, including the Japan Pancreas Society. Recently, some clinicians have used the Mayo Clinic "HISORt Criteria," which rely on *h*istology, *i*maging, *s*erology, *o*rgans of involvement, and *r*espose to corticosteroid therapy.[27,96]

Recently, attention has been given to the concept of stratifying AIP into "Type 1" and "Type 2" autoimmune pancreatitis.[73,90,94] Type 1 is typically used to refer to LPSP, and Type 2 is typically used to refer to IDCP. The expert panel that advocated the use of these terms had some disagreement as to whether these terms should be applied, which features should define each category, and also as to whether the term "autoimmune pancreatitis" should be used with each of these entities; however, it was expressed in their general consensus document (also termed the "Honolulu Consensus Document") that the Type 1 and Type 2 AIP categories will help facilitate further study on these entities.[73] Using a similar definition, a recent study by Deshpande and colleagues[90] found that Type 1 AIP typically includes the cases that have systemic manifestations (ie, sclerosing cholangitis, interstitial nephritis, salivary gland lesions, and lymphadenopathy) and is seen mostly older males with jaundice; and Type 2 AIP is generally limited to the pancreas and is less likely to be associated with a history of alcohol abuse. Type 1 AIP often had an inflamed hypercellular interlobular stroma, and Type 2 had microabscesses and ductal ulceration.

DIABETES MELLITUS

Diabetes mellitus consists of a chronic hyperglycemic state most characteristically because of insufficient insulin production of the pancreas and is typically categorized as Type 1 or 2. Type 1 diabetes mellitus usually occurs in children, who usually require insulin replacement and commonly experience ketoacidosis, and type 2 diabetes more often occurs in adults and can often be treated by diet modification or hypoglycemic medication. Clinically, patients with diabetes usually suffer from hyperglycemia owing to a decreased quantity or effect of insulin; and this is often accompanied by glucosuria, dehydration through water loss, weight loss because of breakdown of body fat, and diabetic coma. Breakdown of body fat leads to circulating free fatty acids, which result in hyperlipidemia and hypercholesterolemia; and these molecules are metabolized into ketone bodies that lead to ketoacidosis. Chronic effects on essentially all organs may result, leading to diabetic retinopathy, diabetic glomerulosclerosis (with Kimmelstiel-Wilson nodules), atherosclerosis, peripheral vascular disease, increased rates of myocardial infarction, and increased rates

of infection.[27,100,101] The pathogenesis of diabetes is complex.[100–108] Type 1 diabetes involves an autoimmune etiology with a genetic predisposition, leading to loss of islet β-cells.[102,105,107,108] The cause of type 2 diabetes is considered to be multifactorial, involving an association with peripheral insulin resistance, impaired islet β-cell function, obesity, and a familial/genetic predisposition.[103,104]

Pathologic findings may not be detectable on the gross level in diabetes. In type 1 diabetes, the pancreas may look normal, particularly if the disease is of recent onset; and after disease has been present for some time, there may be pancreatic atrophy with fibrosis. In type 2 diabetes, there are few if any gross abnormalities.[27,109]

Microscopically, in type 1 diabetes, islets are markedly decreased in size to such an extent that they may be difficult to identify on routine hematoxylin and eosin slides. Islets may consist of small cells in narrow cords in a fibrous stroma, a process termed islet fibrosis. Islets may be involved by an inflammatory infiltrate in a process termed insulitis, a process that may vary in severity from mild or florid. The changes are more prominent in patients younger than 10 years. Beta cells are affected more prominently, and a diminution of beta cells can be demonstrated with immunohistochemistry. There may be interlobular and interacinar fibrosis and exocrine acinar cell atrophy. Large arteries often display atherosclerosis, and smaller arteries may have diabetic microangiopathy. Type 1 diabetes does not typically lead to islet amyloidosis.[27,109,110]

Type 2 diabetes typically has only subtle changes microscopically, commonly displaying no appreciable differences in islet composition when compared with normal pancreatic tissue; however, there may be almost a 50% decrease in islet cell mass, primarily because of a reduction in beta cells. Islet amyloidosis is a common feature in type 2 diabetes (**Fig. 5**); however, it is not entirely pathognomonic because it can be seen in other settings and can even be seen with normal aging. Other characteristics of type 2 diabetes include fatty infiltration of the pancreas and islet fibrosis. Special stains can help identify the amyloid deposits, which stain with thioflavin T and weakly with Congo Red.[27,109,111,112]

EOSINOPHILIC PANCREATITIS

Eosinophilic pancreatitis consists of a prominent infiltration of the pancreas by eosinophils that may sometimes simulate a mass lesion or result in common bile duct obstruction. In its purest form, eosinophilic pancreatitis is rather rare.

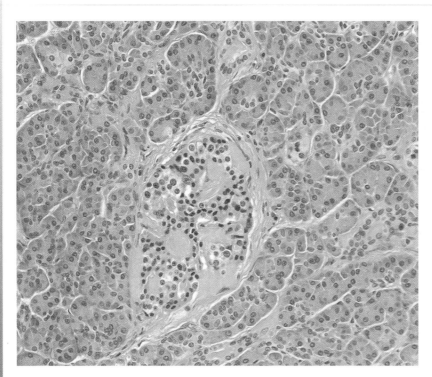

Fig. 5. Diabetes mellitus. This photomicrograph is of the pancreas in a patient with diabetes mellitus, type 2, showing relatively normal lobules and relatively preserved islets with prominent amyloid deposition (H&E).

Prominent eosinophils may be observed in the pancreas in a number of conditions including parasitic infection, hypersensitivity or allergic reactions, such as to drugs or allergens, inflammatory myofibroblastic tumors, or pancreatic allograft rejection. Prominent eosinophils may also be seen in association with pseudocysts in chronic pancreatitis, pancreatic carcinomas, lymphoplasmacytic sclerosing pancreatitis, or the hypereosinophilic syndrome. Patients may have abdominal pain, peripheral eosinophilia, obstructive jaundice, and elevated serum IgE. Eosinophilic infiltrates may be seen in other organs. Eosinophilic syndrome consists of elevated eosinophil count lasting at least 6 months, allergic symptoms, such as rhinitis or asthma, and involvement of multiple organs, such as the gastrointestinal tract, skin, or heart.[27,113–122]

Grossly, the pancreas may be fibrotic and/or enlarged. Microscopically, there is an eosinophilic infiltrate of variable intensity containing eosinophils either localized or diffuse throughout the pancreas. Eosinophils may be seen surrounding acini and ducts and sometimes blood vessels, producing either arteritis or phlebitis. Pseudocysts may be associated with prominent eosinophilic infiltrates in the adjacent pancreatic parenchyma.[113–122]

HEREDITARY PANCREATITIS

Hereditary pancreatitis is characterized by a fibrosing, necroinflammatory disorder beginning in childhood or adolescence, often in the first decade of life. Symptoms are similar to alcoholic pancreatitis: nausea, vomiting, and epigastric pain. Patients may be subject to episodic attacks, which become less severe with age. Laboratory testing may show increased amylase, lipase, increased amylase/creatinine clearance ratio, and sometimes hyperlipidemia, hypercalcemia, and increased serum immunoglobulin concentrations. There is an increased risk of diabetes mellitus, pseudocysts, pancreatic exocrine insufficiency, and abscess formation.[14,27,123–128]

Hereditary pancreatitis is typically thought to be an autosomal dominant disorder showing variable expression and approximately 80% penetrance, affecting women and men equally. Patients have an increased risk of developing pancreatic ductal carcinoma, and overall the lifetime risk is 40% with the highest risk in the 50-year-old to 70-year-old age group. Only about 2% of chronic pancreatitis cases are attributable to hereditary pancreatitis. Certain HLA types are more likely to exhibit hereditary pancreatitis (eg, HLA-B12, HLA-B13, and HLA-Bw40). Many cases are attributable to mutations in the cystic fibrosis transmembrane conductance regulator (CFTR), in the cationic trypsinogen gene (PRSS1), or in the serine protease inhibitor Kazal type 1 (SPINK1). It has been suggested that up to 80% of patients with symptomatic hereditary pancreatitis have an underlying PRSS1 mutation.[14,27,123–128]

The gross and microscopic findings in hereditary pancreatitis are quite similar to those in alcoholic chronic pancreatitis. Rather nonspecific periductal fibrosis and intraductal precipitate accumulation are typically observed. Intraductal calculi and pseudocyst formation can sometimes be seen.[14,27,123–128]

CYSTS AND PSEUDOTUMORS ASSOCIATED WITH PANCREATITIS

A number of non-neoplastic lesions, such as pseudocysts (**Fig. 6**), retention cysts, and lymphoepithelial cysts, may sometimes be present in conjunction with pancreatitis. Pseudocysts typically have a thick wall containing fibrous tissue and granulation tissue without an epithelial lining. They may contain calcification or even ossification (see **Fig. 6**).[14] Neoplastic lesions, including pancreatic intraepithelial neoplasia (PanIN), intraductal papillary mucinous neoplasms (IPMNs), intraductal tubulopapillary neoplasms (IDTNs), and even carcinomas may also be present together with pancreatitis. Many of these entities, especially cystic ones, are covered in more detail in other articles in this issue; therefore, here we mainly focus on those that may present as pseudotumors.

PARADUODENAL ("GROOVE") PANCREATITIS

A form of pancreatitis that occurs in the proximity of the duodenal wall near the minor papilla (**Fig. 7**) is referred to as "paraduodenal pancreatitis." This form of pancreatitis was once often referred to as "groove" pancreatitis. Other names for this disorder included adenomyoma/myoadenomatosis, cystic dystrophy of heterotopic pancreas, pancreatic hamartoma of pancreatic wall, or periampullary or periduodenal wall cyst; however, "paraduodenal" pancreatitis has been commonly used in the recent literature. Inflammation may completely surround the duodenal wall near the minor papilla. Paraduodenal pancreatitis typically involves an area between the pancreas, common bile duct, and duodenum, a feature that gives rise to the term "groove" pancreatitis; the process typically involves the minor papilla, also known as the accessory ampulla. The minor papilla is usually located about 2 cm proximal and somewhat anterior to the ampulla of Vater (also known as the major papilla). The duct of Santorini, a remnant of the embryologic dorsal duct, connects to the duodenal lumen through the accessory ampulla.[20,129–137]

Factors associated with the development of paraduodenal pancreatitis include alcohol abuse, tobacco smoking, and hypertension. Patients present with upper abdominal pain, postprandial vomiting, nausea, and jaundice. A common demographic affected include men in their fifth and sixth decades of life who have a history of alcohol abuse. Hypercalcemia and gallstones are not usually seen. Congenital abnormalities such as pancreatic divisum may play a role in the tendency to develop paraduodenal pancreatitis. Most individuals with paraduodenal pancreatitis are chronic alcoholics, and alcohol, together with congenital abnormalities, may lead to the development of paraduodenal pancreatitis. An important category in the differential diagnosis includes autoimmune disorders. Jaundice, caused by stenosis of the common bile duct, together with the cystic change and mass-forming inflammatory processes, may lead to a suspicion of pancreatic ductal adenocarcinoma; radiographic findings may also mimic a malignancy.[20,129–137]

Grossly, in the duodenal wall there is a thickening and fibrosis, notably around the minor papilla; and there may be cystic changes, which have been likened sometimes to a sieve. Cysts, which have been noted up to 10 cm, typically contain clear fluid and white, granular intracystic material and sometimes even contain stones. The common bile duct may be compressed. Lymph nodes may be enlarged.[20,129–137]

Upon microscopic examination, the duodenal submucosa and muscularis typically has a prominent chronic inflammatory cell infiltrate; and inflammation typically extends into the pancreas. The duodenal mucosa may be ulcerated. There is often a proliferation of smooth muscle cells, which may display a whirling pattern, referred to as a myoid proliferation. Commonly most prominent in the submucosa of the minor papilla, the myoid proliferation often surrounds pancreatic acini, and glandular spaces may undergo cystic dilatation; amidst the myoid proliferation, islets, nerve fibers, and even foci of necrosis may be noted. The myoid cells express smooth muscle actin and other muscle markers, and it has been suggested that they show myofibroblastic differentiation. Acidophilic or amphophilic mucoprotein material may also be seen in ducts; and this material may also sometimes be calcified. Ductal epithelium may be denuded or eroded, leading to cysts that have the appearance of pseudocysts.

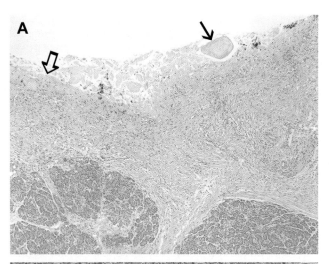

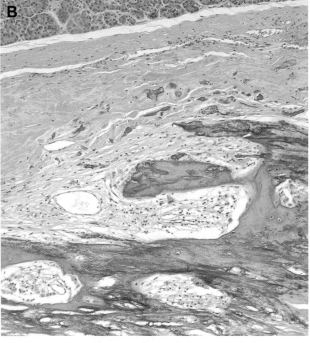

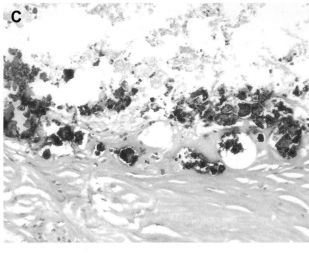

Fig. 6. Pseudocyst. (*A*) Low power (original magnification ×2) of pseudocyst wall showing concretion (*arrow*) and fibrotic wall with granulation-type tissue (*open arrow*). (*B*) Medium power of a pseudocyst wall showing ossification. (*C*) Higher power of pseudocyst contents that have undergone calcification. (All H&E.)

Fig. *7.* Paraduodenal ("groove") pancreatitis. (*A*) At relatively low power, a case of paraduodenal pancreatitis, there is a cyst (*) adjacent to the duodenum (*arrow*) and common bile duct (*open arrow*). (*B*) In a case of paraduodenal pancreatitis, there is prominent Brunner's gland hyperplasia (*arrows*). (All H&E.)

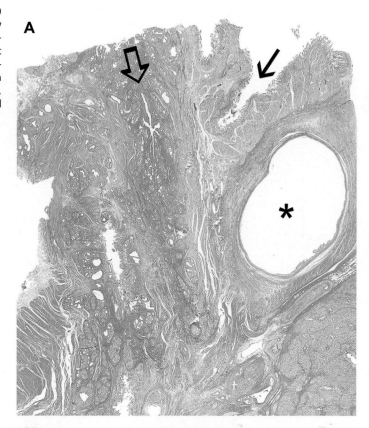

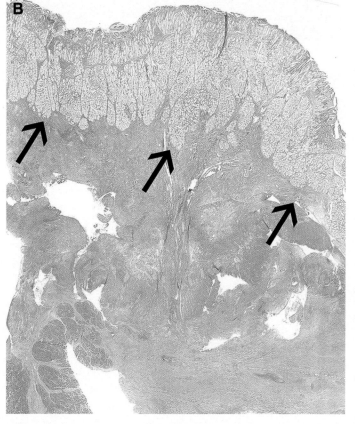

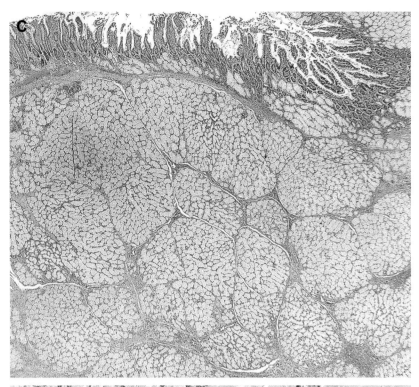

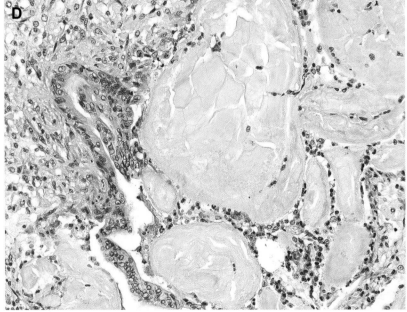

Fig. 7. (*C*) Higher power of the Brunner's gland hyperplasia. (*D*) In a case of paraduodenal pancreatitis, there is a prominent ductal concretion with numerous infiltrating eosinophils.

Ducts may rupture, releasing mucoid material into the surrounding stroma and eliciting a foreign body giant cell reaction and granulation tissue. The inflammatory infiltrate may contain clusters of eosinophils. Brunner's gland hyperplasia may be noted, which may contribute to a thickening of the duodenal wall. A neuronal proliferation can sometimes be seen, sometimes in association with islets and similar in some ways to changes seen in neuromas. It is important to have an appreciation for the microscopic features of paraduodenal pancreatitis because the dilated glands,

Fig. 7. (*E*) A storiform myofibroblastic proliferation can be seen in this case of paraduodenal pancreatitis. (*F*) A focus of abundant eosinophils can be seen adjacent to a nerve in this case of paraduodenal pancreatitis.

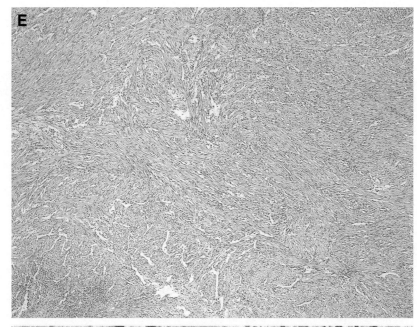

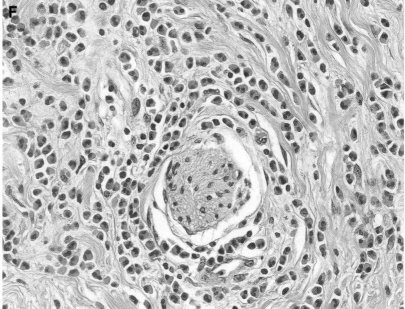

whirling of myoid cells, and neuronal proliferation, may sometimes acquire a pseudoinfiltrative appearance, simulating a neoplasm.[20,129–137]

PANCREATIC "PSEUDOTUMORS"

It seems the vast majority of inflammatory "pseudotumors" arising in the pancreas are associated with autoimmune pancreatitis.[20,88,136] The "inflammatory myofibroblastic" tumors positive for anaplastic lymphoma kinase (ALK) (eg, by immunohistochemistry) do not seem to compose a substantial proportion of pancreatic "pseudotumors." It has been noted that it is important to avoid the term "pseudotumor" when possible, striving to assign a particular diagnostic entity to lesions rather than the nonspecific diagnosis of "pseudotumor."[136] These entities should all be distinguished from malignant lesions, such as pancreatic adenocarcinoma and malignant fibrous histiocytoma.[88] As mentioned previously, paraduodenal pancreatitis can give rise to pseudotumors.[20,136,137]

AMPULLARY ADENOMYOMA

The ampulla of Vater may become impressively thickened, leading to a diagnosis of "pancreas cancer" (also known as a Vaterian adenomyoma, adenomyomatosis, myoepithelial hamartoma, or adenomyomatous hyperplasia).[134,136,138–144] The gross findings, together with clinical and radiologic data, are most diagnostic in this lesion, as the microscopic findings simply show thickened muscle bundles with lobules of peribiliary type ducts. Some cases of this entity may represent ampulla-centric paraduodenal pancreatitis.[136]

HAMARTOMA

Many cases of what have been reported as hamartomas in the literature are likely simply cases of chronic pancreatitis, which result in parenchymal atrophy, yielding disorganized-appearing aggregates of islets, ducts, and atrophic acini. In the strictest sense, true hamartomas of the pancreas do appear to exist. Many of these are found in children and neonates; for example, one well-described entity is the multicystic hamartoma of children.[145,146] Analogous forms appearing in adults are also known as multicystic hamartomas, consisting of solid and cystic lesions with disorganized ductal elements with flattened and cuboidal epithelium with surrounding chronic inflammation. These display predominantly pancreatic polypeptide-secreting endocrine cells without prominent insulin-secreting cells.[136,147] Another type of hamartoma appearing in adults is a solid lesion composed of a spindle-cell stroma containing well-differentiated ducts, resembling a fibroadenoma of the breast. This lesion does not contain islets; however, chromogranin and insulin-positive cells can be found scattered throughout. The spindle cells stain for CD34 and CD117 (c-kit).[136,148]

MISCELLANEOUS CYSTIC PANCREATIC LESIONS OF EXTRAPANCREATIC ORIGIN

Other cystic pancreatic neoplasms unlikely to be confused with the entities presented here include endometriotic cysts, duodenal diverticula, and (congenital) foregut (enteric) cysts. These may be present in conjunction with pancreatitis and awareness of these entities and careful gross and microscopic examination is necessary to appreciate and properly diagnose them. Therefore, these are briefly mentioned here.

Pitfalls
PANCREAS PATHOLOGY

! Care must be given to the interpretation of pancreatic tissue so that changes of chronic pancreatitis are not mistaken for invasive adenocarcinoma.

! Chronic pancreatitis is a rather nonspecific diagnosis, and it is important to adequately classify cases of chronic pancreatitis, such as those associated with IgG4+ plasma cells (ie, in IgG4-associated autoimmune pancreatitis).

Although they may be in close proximity to the pancreas and even outpouch into the pancreas, duodenal diverticula and foregut cysts do not arise in the pancreas proper, and a distinct connection to their site of origin can usually be demonstrated. These cysts may sometimes be associated with pancreatitis.[149] Bundles of smooth muscle can be appreciated in the wall of foregut (or duplication) cysts, and they may contain epithelium of various types, including small intestinal, gastric, squamous, and ciliated columnar.[150,151] Unlike foregut cysts, duodenal diverticula communicate with the duodenal lumen with a mucosal lining continuous with that of the duodenum. The ampulla is a typical site for duodenal diverticula.[33,152] Endometriotic cysts are rather uncommon in the pancreas, and recognition of their characteristic stroma and glands can help distinguish them from pancreatitis.[33,153] Splenic heterotopia is usually composed of typical splenic tissue and is unlikely to be confused with pancreatitis. Lipomatous pseudohypertrophy, also known as lipomatosis or pseudolipomatous hypertrophy, consisting of fatty replacement of pancreatic tissue is a characteristic lesion and usually shows no evidence of pancreatitis.[33,136,154–160]

NEOPLASTIC PREDISPOSITION CAUSED BY INFLAMMATORY LESIONS OF THE PANCREAS

Pancreatic cancer may have an increased incidence in chronic pancreatitis.[16,161,162] Carcinogenesis is likely a multistep process in which factors such as smoking, pancreatitis, and genetic mutations play a role. It has been suggested that mutations in genes such as KRAS, CDKN2A (formerly p16), DPC4, and BRCA2, and microsatellite instability may play a role in the development of pancreatic cancer.[163,164] Alcohol may play a direct role in leading to toxic metabolite activation and cellular organelle damage; for example, alcohol can lead to activation of NF-kappa-B. It is noteworthy to recognize that both chronic pancreatitis and adenocarcinoma have prominent fibrosis, and much pancreatic cancer research has recently focused on the stroma/desmoplastic reaction in the development of pancreatic adenocarcinoma rather than on the biology of the cancer cells themselves. Research has indicated that the pancreatic stellate cell could be an important contributor to the development of pancreatic adenocarcinoma, and there is even evidence to suggest that pancreatic stellate cells accompany cancer cells to metastatic sites.[16]

REFERENCES

1. Sakorafas GH, Tsiotou AG. Etiology and pathogenesis of acute pancreatitis: current concepts. J Clin Gastroenterol 2000;30(4):343–56.

2. Wang GJ, Gao CF, Wei D, et al. Acute pancreatitis: etiology and common pathogenesis. World J Gastroenterol 2009;15(12):1427–30.

3. Ihse I, Lempinen M, Worning H. A clinically based classification system for acute pancreatitis. Summary of the 'Atlanta Classification. Scand J Gastroenterol 1994;29(1):95–6.

4. Ranson JH, Rifkind KM, Roses DF, et al. Prognostic signs and the role of operative management in acute pancreatitis. Surg Gynecol Obstet 1974; 139(1):69–81.

5. Wrobleski DM, Barth MM, Oyen LJ. Necrotizing pancreatitis: pathophysiology, diagnosis, and acute care management. AACN Clin Issues 1999; 10(4):464–77.

6. Lowham A, Lavelle J, Leese T. Mortality from acute pancreatitis. Late septic deaths can be avoided but some early deaths still occur. Int J Pancreatol 1999; 25(2):103–6.

7. Steinberg W, Tenner S. Acute pancreatitis. N Engl J Med 1994;330(17):1198–210.

8. Kloppel G. Acute pancreatitis. Semin Diagn Pathol 2004;21(4):221–6.

9. Pannala R, Kidd M, Modlin IM. Acute pancreatitis: a historical perspective. Pancreas 2009;38(4): 355–66.

10. Sajith KG, Chacko A, Dutta AK. Recurrent acute pancreatitis: clinical profile and an approach to diagnosis. Dig Dis Sci 2010;55(12):3610–6.

11. Golub R, Siddiqi F, Pohl D. Role of antibiotics in acute pancreatitis: a meta-analysis. J Gastrointest Surg 1998;2(6):496–503.

12. Etemad B, Whitcomb DC. Chronic pancreatitis: diagnosis, classification, and new genetic developments. Gastroenterology 2001;120(3):682–707.

13. Uomo G. How far are we from the most accurate classification system for chronic pancreatitis? JOP 2002;3(3):62–5.

14. Kloppel G. Chronic pancreatitis of alcoholic and nonalcoholic origin. Semin Diagn Pathol 2004; 21(4):227–36.

15. Dreiling DA, Koller M. The natural history of alcoholic pancreatitis: update 1985. Mt Sinai J Med 1985;52(5):340–2.

16. Apte M, Pirola R, Wilson J. New insights into alcoholic pancreatitis and pancreatic cancer. J Gastroenterol Hepatol 2009;24(Suppl 3):S51–6.

17. Irving HM, Samokhvalov AV, Rehm J. Alcohol as a risk factor for pancreatitis. A systematic review and meta-analysis. JOP 2009;10(4):387–92.

18. Yadav D, Whitcomb DC. The role of alcohol and smoking in pancreatitis. Nat Rev Gastroenterol Hepatol 2010;7(3):131–45.

19. Law R, Parsi M, Lopez R, et al. Cigarette smoking is independently associated with chronic pancreatitis. Pancreatology 2010;10(1):54–9.

20. Kloppel G. Chronic pancreatitis, pseudotumors and other tumor-like lesions. Mod Pathol 2007; 20(Suppl 1):S113–31.

21. O'Sullivan JN, Nobrega FT, Morlock CG, et al. Acute and chronic pancreatitis in Rochester, Minnesota, 1940 to 1969. Gastroenterology 1972; 62(3):373–9.

22. Morris-Stiff G, Teli M, Jardine N, et al. CA19-9 antigen levels can distinguish between benign and malignant pancreaticobiliary disease. Hepatobiliary Pancreat Dis Int 2009;8(6):620–6.

23. Raghu MG, Wig JD, Kochhar R, et al. Lung complications in acute pancreatitis. JOP 2007;8(2):177–85.

24. Chen WX, Zhang WF, Li B, et al. Clinical manifestations of patients with chronic pancreatitis. Hepatobiliary Pancreat Dis Int 2006;5(1):133–7.

25. Lanitis S, Sivakumar S, Zaman N, et al. Recurrent acute pancreatitis as the first and sole presentation of undiagnosed primary hyperparathyroidism. Ann R Coll Surg Engl 2010;92(2):W29–31.

26. Sitges-Serra A, Alonso M, de Lecea C, et al. Pancreatitis and hyperparathyroidism. Br J Surg 1988;75(2):158–60.

27. Wenig BM, Heffess CS. Inflammatory, infectious, and other non-neoplastic disorders of the pancreas. In: Odze RD, editor. Surgical pathology of the GI tract, liver, biliary tract, and pancreas. 2nd edition. Philadelphia: Saunders Elsevier; 2009. p. 878–908.

28. Hyland C, Kheir SM, Kashlan MB. Frozen section diagnosis of pancreatic carcinoma: a prospective study of 64 biopsies. Am J Surg Pathol 1981;5(2): 179–91.

29. Adsay NV, Bandyopadhyay S, Basturk O, et al. Chronic pancreatitis or pancreatic ductal adenocarcinoma? Semin Diagn Pathol 2004;21(4):268–76.

30. Ballian N, Hu M, Liu SH, et al. Proliferation, hyperplasia, neogenesis, and neoplasia in the islets of Langerhans. Pancreas 2007;35(3):199–206.

31. Bartow SA, Mukai K, Rosai J. Pseudoneoplastic proliferation of endocrine cells in pancreatic fibrosis. Cancer 1981;47(11):2627–33.

32. Sangueza O, Wei J, Isales CM. Pancreatic fibrosis with islet cell pseudoneoplastic proliferation as a cause of hypoglycemia. Ann Intern Med 1997; 127(11):1042–3.

33. Hruban RH, Pitman MB, Klimstra DS. Tumors of the pancreas. Washington, DC: American Registry of Pathology; 2007.

34. Bommer G, Friedl U, Heitz PU, et al. Pancreatic PP cell distribution and hyperplasia. Immunocytochemical morphology in the normal human pancreas, in chronic pancreatitis and pancreatic carcinoma. Virchows Arch A Pathol Anat Histol 1980;387(3):319–31.

35. Mahurkar S, Reddy DN, Rao GV, et al. Genetic mechanisms underlying the pathogenesis of tropical calcific pancreatitis. World J Gastroenterol 2009;15(3):264–9.

36. Witt H, Bhatia E. Genetic aspects of tropical calcific pancreatitis. Rev Endocr Metab Disord 2008;9(3): 213–26.

37. Tandon RK. Tropical pancreatitis. J Gastroenterol 2007;42(Suppl 17):141–7.

38. Barman KK, Premalatha G, Mohan V. Tropical chronic pancreatitis. Postgrad Med J 2003; 79(937):606–15.

39. Mohan V, Premalatha G, Pitchumoni CS. Tropical chronic pancreatitis: an update. J Clin Gastroenterol 2003;36(4):337–46.

40. Bhatia E, Choudhuri G, Sikora SS, et al. Tropical calcific pancreatitis: strong association with SPINK1 trypsin inhibitor mutations. Gastroenterology 2002;123(4):1020–5.

41. Chandak GR, Idris MM, Reddy DN, et al. Mutations in the pancreatic secretory trypsin inhibitor gene (PSTI/SPINK1) rather than the cationic trypsinogen gene (PRSS1) are significantly associated with tropical calcific pancreatitis. J Med Genet 2002; 39(5):347–51.

42. Parenti DM, Steinberg W, Kang P. Infectious causes of acute pancreatitis. Pancreas 1996; 13(4):356–71.

43. Dassopoulos T, Ehrenpreis ED. Acute pancreatitis in human immunodeficiency virus-infected patients: a review. Am J Med 1999;107(1):78–84.

44. Cappell MS. The pancreas in AIDS. Gastroenterol Clin North Am 1997;26(2):337–65.

45. Parithivel VS, Yousuf AM, Albu E, et al. Predictors of the severity of acute pancreatitis in patients with HIV infection or AIDS. Pancreas 1999;19(2):133–6.

46. Manocha AP, Sossenheimer M, Martin SP, et al. Prevalence and predictors of severe acute pancreatitis in patients with acquired immune deficiency syndrome (AIDS). Am J Gastroenterol 1999; 94(3):784–9.

47. Hviid A, Rubin S, Muhlemann K. Mumps. Lancet 2008;371(9616):932–44.

48. Huber S, Ramsingh AI. Coxsackievirus-induced pancreatitis. Viral Immunol 2004;17(3):358–69.

49. Ramsingh AI. Coxsackieviruses and pancreatitis. Front Biosci 1997;2:e53–62.

50. Franco-Paredes C, Leonard M, Jurado R, et al. Tuberculosis of the pancreas: report of two cases and review of the literature. Am J Med Sci 2002; 323(1):54–8.

51. Riedlinger WF, Lairmore TC, Balfe DM, et al. Tumefactive necrobiotic granulomas (nodulosis) of the pancreas in an adult with long-standing rheumatoid arthritis. Int J Surg Pathol 2005;13(2):207–10.

52. Mackrell PJ, Lee K, Garcia N, et al. Pancreatitis secondary to Ascaris lumbricoides infestation. Surgery 2001;129(4):511–2.

53. Kim YH. Extrahepatic cholangiocarcinoma associated with clonorchiasis: CT evaluation. Abdom Imaging 2003;28(1):68–71.

54. Kim YH. Pancreatitis in association with Clonorchis sinensis infestation: CT evaluation. AJR Am J Roentgenol 1999;172(5):1293–6.

55. Lim JH, Ko YT. Clonorchiasis of the pancreas. Clin Radiol 1990;41(3):195–8.

56. Chan PH, Teoh TB. The pathology of Clonorchis sinensis infestation of the pancreas. J Pathol Bacteriol 1967;93(1):185–9.

57. Perez-Jorge EV, Burdette SD. Association between acute pancreatitis and Strongyloides stercoralis. South Med J 2008;101(7):771–2.

58. Pijls NH, Yap SH, Rosenbusch G, et al. Pancreatic mass due to Strongyloides stercoralis infection: an unusual manifestation. Pancreas 1986;1(1):90–3.

59. Hofman P, Michiels JF, Mondain V, et al. [Acute toxoplasmic pancreatitis. An unusual cause of death in AIDS]. Gastroenterol Clin Biol 1994; 18(10):895–7 [in French].

60. Sturmer J, Becker V. Granulomatous pancreatitis—granulomas in chronic pancreatitis. Virchows Arch A Pathol Anat Histopathol 1987;410(4):327–38.

61. Boruchowicz A, Vandermolen P, Colombel JF. Granulomatous pancreatitis: Crohn's disease or sarcoidosis? Gastroenterology 1996;110(1):321–2.

62. Boruchowicz A, Wallaert B, Cortot A, et al. Idiopathic acute pancreatitis and sarcoidosis. Gastroenterol Clin Biol 1995;19(4):439–41.

63. Bacal D, Hoshal VL Jr, Schaldenbrand JD, et al. Sarcoidosis of the pancreas: case report and review of the literature. Am Surg 2000;66(7):675–8.

64. Caceres M, Sabbaghian MS, Braud R, et al. Pancreatic sarcoidosis: unusual presentation resembling a periampullary malignancy. Curr Surg 2006;63(3):179–85.

65. Deshpande V, Chicano S, Finkelberg D, et al. Autoimmune pancreatitis: a systemic immune complex mediated disease. Am J Surg Pathol 2006;30(12): 1537–45.

66. Deshpande V, Mino-Kenudson M, Brugge W, et al. Autoimmune pancreatitis: more than just a pancreatic disease? A contemporary review of its pathology. Arch Pathol Lab Med 2005;129(9): 1148–54.

67. Deshpande V, Mino-Kenudson M, Brugge WR, et al. Endoscopic ultrasound guided fine needle aspiration biopsy of autoimmune pancreatitis: diagnostic criteria and pitfalls. Am J Surg Pathol 2005; 29(11):1464–71.

68. Finkelberg DL, Sahani D, Deshpande V, et al. Autoimmune pancreatitis. N Engl J Med 2006;355(25): 2670–6.

69. Ball WP, Baggenstoss AH, Bargen JA. Pancreatic lesions associated with chronic ulcerative colitis. Arch Pathol (Chic) 1950;50(3):347–58.

70. Sarles H, Sarles JC, Camatte R, et al. Observations on 205 confirmed cases of acute pancreatitis, recurring pancreatitis, and chronic pancreatitis. Gut 1965;6(6):545–59.

71. Sarles H, Sarles JC, Muratore R, et al. Chronic inflammatory sclerosis of the pancreas—an autonomous pancreatic disease? Am J Dig Dis 1961;6: 688–98.

72. Yoshida K, Toki F, Takeuchi T, et al. Chronic pancreatitis caused by an autoimmune abnormality. Proposal of the concept of autoimmune pancreatitis. Dig Dis Sci 1995;40(7):1561–8.

73. Chari ST, Kloeppel G, Zhang L, et al. Histopathologic and clinical subtypes of autoimmune pancreatitis: the Honolulu consensus document. Pancreas 2010;39(5):549–54.

74. Deshpande V, Sainani NI, Chung RT, et al. IgG4-associated cholangitis: a comparative histological and immunophenotypic study with primary sclerosing cholangitis on liver biopsy material. Mod Pathol 2009;22(10):1287–95.

75. Wang WL, Farris AB, Lauwers GY, et al. Autoimmune pancreatitis-related cholecystitis: a morphologically and immunologically distinctive form of lymphoplasmacytic sclerosing cholecystitis. Histopathology 2009;54(7):829–36.

76. Cornell LD, Chicano SL, Deshpande V, et al. Pseudotumors due to IgG4 immune-complex tubulointerstitial nephritis associated with autoimmune pancreatocentric disease. Am J Surg Pathol 2007;31(10):1586–97.

77. Geyer JT, Ferry JA, Harris NL, et al. Chronic sclerosing sialadenitis (Kuttner tumor) is an IgG4-associated disease. Am J Surg Pathol 2010;34(2): 202–10.

78. Shrestha B, Sekiguchi H, Colby TV, et al. Distinctive pulmonary histopathology with increased IgG4-positive plasma cells in patients with autoimmune pancreatitis: report of 6 and 12 cases with similar histopathology. Am J Surg Pathol 2009;33(10): 1450–62.

79. Mino-Kenudson M, Lauwers GY. Histopathology of autoimmune pancreatitis: recognized features and unsolved issues. J Gastrointest Surg 2005;9(1): 6–10.

80. Farris AB 3rd, Lauwers GY, Deshpande V. Autoimmune pancreatitis-related diabetes: quantitative analysis of endocrine islet cells and inflammatory infiltrate. Virchows Arch 2010;457(3):329–36.

81. Hamano H, Kawa S, Horiuchi A, et al. High serum IgG4 concentrations in patients with sclerosing pancreatitis. N Engl J Med 2001;344(10): 732–8.

82. Okazaki K, Uchida K, Ohana M, et al. Autoimmune-related pancreatitis is associated with autoantibodies and a Th1/Th2-type cellular immune response. Gastroenterology 2000;118(3):573–81.

83. Uchida K, Okazaki K, Konishi Y, et al. Clinical analysis of autoimmune-related pancreatitis. Am J Gastroenterol 2000;95(10):2788–94.

84. Ito T, Nakano I, Koyanagi S, et al. Autoimmune pancreatitis as a new clinical entity. Three cases of autoimmune pancreatitis with effective steroid therapy. Dig Dis Sci 1997;42(7):1458–68.

85. Uchida K, Satoi S, Miyoshi H, et al. Inflammatory pseudotumors of the pancreas and liver with infiltration of IgG4-positive plasma cells. Intern Med 2007;46(17):1409–12.

86. Uchida K, Okazaki K, Asada M, et al. Case of chronic pancreatitis involving an autoimmune mechanism that extended to retroperitoneal fibrosis. Pancreas 2003;26(1):92–4.

87. Chutaputti A, Burrell MI, Boyer JL. Pseudotumor of the pancreas associated with retroperitoneal fibrosis: a dramatic response to corticosteroid therapy. Am J Gastroenterol 1995;90(7):1155–8.

88. Mizukami H, Yajima N, Wada R, et al. Pancreatic malignant fibrous histiocytoma, inflammatory myofibroblastic tumor, and inflammatory pseudotumor related to autoimmune pancreatitis: characterization and differential diagnosis. Virchows Arch 2006;448(5):552–60.

89. Nonomura A, Minato H, Shimizu K, et al. Hepatic hilar inflammatory pseudotumor mimicking cholangiocarcinoma with cholangitis and phlebitis—a variant of primary sclerosing cholangitis? Pathol Res Pract 1997;193(7):519–25 [discussion: 526].

90. Deshpande V, Gupta R, Sainani N, et al. Subclassification of autoimmune pancreatitis: a histologic classification with clinical significance. Am J Surg Pathol 2011;35(1):26–35.

91. Kloppel G, Sipos B, Zamboni G, et al. Autoimmune pancreatitis: histo- and immunopathological features. J Gastroenterol 2007;42(Suppl 18):28–31.

92. Notohara K, Burgart LJ, Yadav D, et al. Idiopathic chronic pancreatitis with periductal lymphoplasmacytic infiltration: clinicopathologic features of 35 cases. Am J Surg Pathol 2003;27(8):1119–27.

93. Zamboni G, Luttges J, Capelli P, et al. Histopathological features of diagnostic and clinical relevance in autoimmune pancreatitis: a study on 53 resection specimens and 9 biopsy specimens. Virchows Arch 2004;445(6):552–63.

94. Park DH, Kim MH, Chari ST. Recent advances in autoimmune pancreatitis. Gut 2009;58(12):1680–9.

95. Zhang L, Notohara K, Levy MJ, et al. IgG4-positive plasma cell infiltration in the diagnosis of autoimmune pancreatitis. Mod Pathol 2007;20(1):23–8.

96. Chari ST. Diagnosis of autoimmune pancreatitis using its five cardinal features: introducing the Mayo Clinic's HISORt criteria. J Gastroenterol 2007;42(Suppl 18):39–41.

97. Kwon S, Kim MH, Choi EK. The diagnostic criteria for autoimmune chronic pancreatitis: it is time to make a consensus. Pancreas 2007; 34(3):279–86.

98. Kojima M, Sipos B, Klapper W, et al. Autoimmune pancreatitis: frequency, IgG4 expression, and clonality of T and B cells. Am J Surg Pathol 2007;31(4): 521–8.

99. Sepehr A, Mino-Kenudson M, Ogawa F, et al. IgG4+ to IgG+ plasma cells ratio of ampulla can help differentiate autoimmune pancreatitis from other "mass forming" pancreatic lesions. Am J Surg Pathol 2008;32(12):1770–9.

100. Flyvbjerg A. Diabetic angiopathy, the complement system and the tumor necrosis factor superfamily. Nat Rev Endocrinol 2010;6(2):94–101.

101. Atkins RC, Zimmet P. Diabetes: diabetic kidney disease: act now or pay later. Nat Rev Nephrol 2010;6(3):134–6.

102. Atkinson MA, Gianani R. The pancreas in human type 1 diabetes: providing new answers to age-old questions. Curr Opin Endocrinol Diabetes Obes 2009;16(4):279–85.

103. O'Rahilly S, Barroso I, Wareham NJ. Genetic factors in type 2 diabetes: the end of the beginning? Science 2005;307(5708):370–3.

104. Lazar MA. How obesity causes diabetes: not a tall tale. Science 2005;307(5708):373–5.

105. Burn P. Type 1 diabetes. Nat Rev Drug Discov 2010;9(3):187–8.

106. Frank RN. Diabetic retinopathy. N Engl J Med 2004; 350(1):48–58.

107. Concannon P, Rich SS, Nepom GT. Genetics of type 1A diabetes. N Engl J Med 2009;360(16): 1646–54.

108. Davidson A, Diamond B. Autoimmune diseases. N Engl J Med 2001;345(5):340–50.

109. Kloppel G, Gepts W, In't Veld PA. Morphology of the pancreas in normal and diabetic states.

In: Alberti KG, DeFronzo RA, Keen H, et al, editors, International textbook of diabetes mellitus, vol. 1. New York: John Wiley and Sons Ltd.; 1992. p. 224–59.

110. Junker K, Egeberg J, Kromann H, et al. An autopsy study of the islets of Langerhans in acute-onset juvenile diabetes mellitus. Acta Pathol Microbiol Scand A 1977;85(5):699–706.

111. Westermark P, Johnson KH. The polypeptide hormone-derived amyloid forms: nonspecific alterations or signs of abnormal peptide-processing? APMIS 1988;96(6):475–83.

112. Bell ET. Hyalinization of the islets of Langerhans in nondiabetic individuals. Am J Pathol 1959;35(4): 801–5.

113. Abraham SC, Leach S, Yeo CJ, et al. Eosinophilic pancreatitis and increased eosinophils in the pancreas. Am J Surg Pathol 2003;27(3):334–42.

114. Barthet M, Hastier P, Buckley MJ, et al. Eosinophilic pancreatitis mimicking pancreatic neoplasia: EUS and ERCP findings—is nonsurgical diagnosis possible? Pancreas 1998;17(4):419–22.

115. Maeshima A, Murakami H, Sadakata H, et al. Eosinophilic gastroenteritis presenting with acute pancreatitis. J Med 1997;28(3–4):265–72.

116. Bastid C, Sahel J, Choux R, et al. Eosinophilic pancreatitis: report of a case. Pancreas 1990; 5(1):104–7.

117. Flejou JF, Potet F, Bernades P. [Eosinophilic pancreatitis: a rare manifestation of digestive allergy?] Gastroenterol Clin Biol 1989;13(8–9): 731–3 [in French].

118. Euscher E, Vaswani K, Frankel W. Eosinophilic pancreatitis: a rare entity that can mimic a pancreatic neoplasm. Ann Diagn Pathol 2000;4(6):379–85.

119. Rakesh K, Banerjee R, Gupta R, et al. Eosinophilic pancreatitis with pseudocyst. Indian J Gastroenterol 2007;26(3):136–7.

120. Cay A, Imamoglu M, Cobanoglu U. Eosinophilic pancreatitis mimicking pancreatic neoplasia. Can J Gastroenterol 2006;20(5):361–4.

121. Stevens T, Mackey R, Falk GW, et al. Eosinophilic pancreatitis presenting as a pancreatic mass with obstructive jaundice. Gastrointest Endosc 2006; 63(3):525–7.

122. Le Connie D, Nguyen H. Eosinophilic gastroenteritis, ascites, and pancreatitis: a case report and review of the literature. South Med J 2004;97(9):905–6.

123. Rosendahl J, Bodeker H, Mossner J, et al. Hereditary chronic pancreatitis. Orphanet J Rare Dis 2007;2:1.

124. Whitcomb DC. Hereditary pancreatitis: a model for understanding the genetic basis of acute and chronic pancreatitis. Pancreatology 2001;1(6): 565–70.

125. Howes N, Lerch MM, Greenhalf W, et al. Clinical and genetic characteristics of hereditary pancreatitis in

Europe. Clin Gastroenterol Hepatol 2004;2(3): 252–61.

126. Teich N, Rosendahl J, Toth M, et al. Mutations of human cationic trypsinogen (PRSS1) and chronic pancreatitis. Hum Mutat 2006;27(8):721–30.

127. Keiles S, Kammesheidt A. Identification of CFTR, PRSS1, and SPINK1 mutations in 381 patients with pancreatitis. Pancreas 2006;33(3):221–7.

128. Tzetis M, Kaliakatsos M, Fotoulaki M, et al. Contribution of the CFTR gene, the pancreatic secretory trypsin inhibitor gene (SPINK1) and the cationic trypsinogen gene (PRSS1) to the etiology of recurrent pancreatitis. Clin Genet 2007;71(5):451–7.

129. Adsay NV, Zamboni G. Paraduodenal pancreatitis: a clinico-pathologically distinct entity unifying "cystic dystrophy of heterotopic pancreas," "para-duodenal wall cyst," and "groove pancreatitis." Semin Diagn Pathol 2004;21(4):247–54.

130. Chatelain D, Vibert E, Yzet T, et al. Groove pancreatitis and pancreatic heterotopia in the minor duodenal papilla. Pancreas 2005;30(4):e92–5.

131. Balakrishnan V, Chatni S, Radhakrishnan L, et al. Groove pancreatitis: a case report and review of literature. JOP 2007;8(5):592–7.

132. Flejou JF, Potet F, Molas G, et al. Cystic dystrophy of the gastric and duodenal wall developing in heterotopic pancreas: an unrecognised entity. Gut 1993;34(3):343–7.

133. McFaul CD, Vitone LJ, Campbell F, et al. Pancreatic hamartoma. Pancreatology 2004;4(6):533–7 [discussion: 537–8].

134. Bill K, Belber JP, Carson JW. Adenomyoma (pancreatic heterotopia) of the duodenum producing common bile duct obstruction. Gastrointest Endosc 1982;28(3):182–4.

135. Casetti L, Bassi C, Salvia R, et al. "Paraduodenal" pancreatitis: results of surgery on 58 consecutives patients from a single institution. World J Surg 2009;33(12):2664–9.

136. Adsay NV, Basturk O, Klimstra DS, et al. Pancreatic pseudotumors: non-neoplastic solid lesions of the pancreas that clinically mimic pancreas cancer. Semin Diagn Pathol 2004;21(4):260–7.

137. Zamboni G, Capelli P, Scarpa A, et al. Nonneoplastic mimickers of pancreatic neoplasms. Arch Pathol Lab Med 2009;133(3):439–53.

138. Noun R, Sayegh R, Tohme-Noun C, et al. Extracystic biliary carcinoma associated with anomalous pancreaticobiliary junction and cysts. J Hepatobiliary Pancreat Surg 2006;13(6):577–9.

139. Bedirli A, Patiroglu TE, Sozuer EM, et al. Periampullary adenomyoma: report of two cases. Surg Today 2002;32(11):1016–8.

140. Handra-Luca A, Terris B, Couvelard A, et al. Adenomyoma and adenomyomatous hyperplasia of the Vaterian system: clinical, pathological, and new immunohistochemical features of 13 cases. Mod Pathol 2003;16(6):530–6.

141. Kayahara M, Ohta T, Kitagawa H, et al. Adenomyomatosis of the papilla of Vater: a case illustrating diagnostic difficulties. Dig Surg 2001;18(2):139–42.

142. Venu RP, Rolny P, Geenen JE, et al. Ampullary hamartoma: endoscopic diagnosis and treatment. Gastroenterology 1991;100(3):795–8.

143. Ulich TR, Kollin M, Simmons GE, et al. Adenomyoma of the papilla of Vater. Arch Pathol Lab Med 1987;111(4):388–90.

144. Dardinski VJ. Inflammatory adenomatoid hyperplasia of the major duodenal papilla in man. Am J Pathol 1931;7(5):519–22 511.

145. Flaherty MJ, Benjamin DR. Multicystic pancreatic hamartoma: a distinctive lesion with immunohistochemical and ultrastructural study. Hum Pathol 1992;23(11):1309–12.

146. Burt TB, Condon VR, Matlak ME. Fetal pancreatic hamartoma. Pediatr Radiol 1983;13(5):287–9.

147. Pauser U, Kosmahl M, Kruslin B, et al. Pancreatic solid and cystic hamartoma in adults: characterization of a new tumorous lesion. Am J Surg Pathol 2005;29(6):797–800.

148. Pauser U, da Silva MT, Placke J, et al. Cellular hamartoma resembling gastrointestinal stromal tumor: a solid tumor of the pancreas expressing c-kit (CD117). Mod Pathol 2005;18(9):1211–6.

149. Lavine JE, Harrison M, Heyman MB. Gastrointestinal duplications causing relapsing pancreatitis in children. Gastroenterology 1989;97(6):1556–8.

150. Demetriadis D, Ververidis M, Papathanasiou D, et al. Pancreatitis due to cystic duodenal duplication in a 12-year-old child. Eur J Pediatr Surg 1997;7(2):109–11.

151. Kohzaki S, Fukuda T, Fujimoto T, et al. Case report: ciliated foregut cyst of the pancreas mimicking teratomatous tumour. Br J Radiol 1994;67(798):601–4.

152. Adsay NV, Hasteh F, Cheng JD, et al. Lymphoepithelial cysts of the pancreas: a report of 12 cases and a review of the literature. Mod Pathol 2002; 15(5):492–501.

153. Marchevsky AM, Zimmerman MJ, Aufses AH Jr, et al. Endometrial cyst of the pancreas. Gastroenterology 1984;86(6):1589–91.

154. Halpert B, Alden ZA. Accessory spleens in or at the tail of the pancreas. A survey of 2,700 additional necropsies. Arch Pathol 1964;77:652–4.

155. Cahalane SF, Kiesselbach N. The significance of the accessory spleen. J Pathol 1970;100(2):139–44.

156. Morohoshi T, Hamamoto T, Kunimura T, et al. Epidermoid cyst derived from an accessory spleen in the pancreas. A case report with literature survey. Acta Pathol Jpn 1991;41(12):916–21.

157. Adsay NV, Hasteh F, Cheng JD, et al. Squamous-lined cysts of the pancreas: lymphoepithelial cysts, dermoid cysts (teratomas), and accessory-splenic

epidermoid cysts. Semin Diagn Pathol 2000;17(1): 56–65.

158. Tateyama H, Tada T, Murase T, et al. Lymphoepithelial cyst and epidermoid cyst of the accessory spleen in the pancreas. Mod Pathol 1998;11(12):1171–7.

159. Servais EL, Sarkaria IS, Solomon GJ, et al. Giant epidermoid cyst within an intrapancreatic accessory spleen mimicking a cystic neoplasm of the pancreas: case report and review of the literature. Pancreas 2008;36(1):98–100.

160. Mortele KJ, Mortele B, Silverman SG. CT features of the accessory spleen. AJR Am J Roentgenol 2004;183(6):1653–7.

161. Lowenfels AB, Maisonneuve P, Cavallini G, et al. Pancreatitis and the risk of pancreatic cancer. International Pancreatitis Study Group. N Engl J Med 1993;328(20):1433–7.

162. Michaud DS. Epidemiology of pancreatic cancer. Minerva Chir 2004;59(2):99–111.

163. Cottliar AS, Fundia AF, Moran C, et al. Evidence of chromosome instability in chronic pancreatitis. J Exp Clin Cancer Res 2000;19(4):513–7.

164. Gerdes B, Ramaswamy A, Kersting M, et al. p16(INK4a) alterations in chronic pancreatitis—indicator for high-risk lesions for pancreatic cancer. Surgery 2001;129(4):490–7.

CYTOLOGY OF THE PANCREAS: A PRACTICAL REVIEW FOR CYTOPATHOLOGISTS

Michelle Reid, MBBS

KEYWORDS

• Pancreas • Cytopathology • Fine-needle aspiration

ABSTRACT

Pancreatic cytopathology plays a critical role in the management of patients with cystic and solid pancreatic masses. The frequency of pancreatic fine-needle aspiration continues to increase and general surgical pathologists and cytopathologists need to be aware of the most commonly encountered entities as well as the pitfalls associated with gastrointestinal tract contaminants in endoscopic ultrasound-guided fine-needle aspiration. This article focuses on the most commonly encountered pancreatic lesions and the importance of correlation of cytologic features with clinical, radiologic, and ancillary studies for accurate diagnosis.

OVERVIEW

Cytologic evaluation of the pancreas is usually performed to evaluate suspicious pancreatic masses and cysts. The most common method of sampling is by fine-needle aspiration biopsy (FNAB), of which there are 2 types: percutaneous aspiration biopsy and endoscopic ultrasound-guided biopsy (EUS).[1] Percutaneous pancreatic FNAB was once the most commonly used method. It is usually performed by a radiologist under computerized tomography (CT) guidance[2] or by transabdominal ultrasound.[3] EUS-FNAB has recently emerged as a more popular alternative to percutaneous FNAB.[4] Such biopsies are performed by a gastroenterologist who places an echoendoscope against the stomach or duodenal wall to obtain a high-resolution image of the area of interest in the pancreas. EUS-FNAB has been growing in frequency because of its increased ability to detect and resolve subcentimeter (0.5 cm) lesions.[1,5] CT-guided FNAB more frequently misses these subcentimeter lesions. EUS-FNAB has the additional advantage of being able to simultaneously diagnose and stage patients by identifying local metastases and invasion of adjacent structures.[1,4] It also allows the real-time visualization of the tip of the needle during the biopsy process.[1,6] Therefore, it is now considered to be the primary, most cost-effective and sensitive modality for investigating pancreatic masses.[1,4,7]

Pancreatic duct and biliary duct brushings are also performed to investigate pancreatobiliary tract pathology. These are usually done endoscopically in conjunction with endoscopic retrograde cholangio-pancreatography or by percutaneous trans-hepatic cholangiography.[1] Pancreatic duct and biliary tract cytopathology will not be discussed in this article.

The interpretation of pancreatic cytopathology is a challenging and difficult task for cytopathologists in general and for general surgical pathologists in particular. Cytologic diagnosis of pancreatic lesions does not depend on morphology alone and must incorporate the analysis of pertinent clinical, radiologic, and ancillary data.[5]

The initial assessment of pancreatic lesions is based on radiologic findings. Most lesions are

Department of Pathology, Emory University Hospital, 1364 Clifton Road NE, Room H190, Atlanta, GA 30322, USA
E-mail address: michelle.reid@emory.edu

Surgical Pathology 4 (2011) 651–691
doi:10.1016/j.path.2011.03.006
1875-9181/11/$ – see front matter © 2011 Elsevier Inc. All rights reserved.

solid, cystic, or mixed. Solid lesions are more common than cystic lesions. The most common solid and cystic pancreatic lesions and neoplasms are described in **Table 1**. Ductal adenocarcinoma accounts for most (90%) solid lesions, followed by chronic pancreatitis, pancreatic endocrine neoplasms (PEN), acinar cell carcinoma, pancreatoblastoma, and metastatic tumors.[5] Most cystic lesions are benign[8] and pancreatic pseudocysts account for most (75%) of these.[1] Pancreatic pseudocysts must be distinguished from neoplastic mucinous cysts, lymphoepithelial cysts, serous cysts, and solid neoplasms with cystic degeneration.

ACCURACY OF PANCREATIC CYTOPATHOLOGY

The sensitivity of pancreatic FNAB for detecting malignancy ranges from 86% to 98% for percutaneous FNAB[9–12] versus 75% to 94% for EUS-FNAB.[1,6] The specificity for both percutaneous and EUS-guided FNAB approaches 100%.[1,5,6] The accuracy of diagnosis is improved by on-site evaluation of adequacy by a cytotechnologist or cytopathologist.[1,4–6] False-positive and false-negative results do occur and are related to sampling and interpretation errors. False-negative interpretations are more common and often occur because of misinterpretation of a well-differentiated ductal carcinoma as benign ductal cells.[1] False-positive results are less common and result when pancreatitis-related reactive atypia is overinterpreted as being malignant. There are a few minor and major complications of pancreatic FNAB. Minor complications include vasovagal reactions, pain, and minor

hemorrhage.[1] Major complications include acute pancreatitis,[13] which is seen in 1% to 3% of cases (and may result in death[14]), massive hemorrhage, perforation,[13] and sepsis.[1,4] Percutaneous pancreatic FNAB has been associated with needle tract seeding, whereas EUS-FNAB has not.[15]

SAMPLE EVALUATION

A cytopathologist should ideally be present at the time of FNAB to immediately evaluate specimens for adequacy. The rapid interpretation of smears increases diagnostic yield and allows for the immediate determination of the need for ancillary studies.[4,16] In addition, the cytopathologist's presence ensures that critical clinical and radiologic information is accurately conveyed. The aspirated sample should be deposited and immediately smeared onto one or more slides using another glass slide. Air-dried and alcohol-fixed slides should then be prepared for evaluation. Air-dried slides can be stained with the Diff-Quik or hemacolor stain and used for immediate on-site evaluation of adequacy. Alcohol-fixed slides can be stained at a later time with the Papanicolaou and hematoxylin and eosin stains. It is also extremely important to collect needle rinses at the time of the FNAB, as these can be used to make cell blocks on which immunohistochemical stains can be performed to differentiate ductal adenocarcinoma from its look-alikes (including pancreatic endocrine neoplasms, acinar cell carcinoma, and solid-pseudopapillary neoplasms). After review of Diff-Quik smears, one can determine the need for ancillary studies, such as flow cytometry (if lymphoma is suspected), culture (if infection is suspected), electron microscopy, and cyst fluid analysis.

The fluid collected from cystic lesions can be submitted for multiple studies at the time of FNAB. These include pancreatic enzymes (amylase, lipase, and leukocyte esterase), tumor markers, viscosity, and molecular markers (K-ras, tumor suppressor genes, microsatellite markers, allelic loss).[1] Cyst fluid amylase, lipase, and leukocyte esterase levels are usually high in pancreatic pseudocysts and low in neoplastic cysts.[17] The tumor markers that can be performed on cyst fluid include carcinoembryonic antigen (CEA), cancer antigen 125 (CA125), CA19.9, CA72-4, and CA15-3. Of these, CEA is the most accurate at distinguishing between benign cysts and mucinous cystic lesions.[1] Low CEA values (<5 ng/mL)[1,5] are typical of pseudocysts[8] and serous cystadenomas.[1,5,18] High CEA values of greater than 200 ng/mL are more predictive of mucinous neoplasms,[5] and

Gross Appearance	Neoplasm
Solid	Ductal adenocarcinoma
	Pancreatic endocrine neoplasm
	Acinar cell carcinoma
	Pancreatoblastoma
Cystic - high risk	Intraductal papillary mucinous neoplasm
	Mucinous cystic neoplasm
Cystic - low risk	Pseudocyst
	Lymphoepithelial cyst
	Serous cystadenoma
Mixed solid and cystic	Solid-pseudopapillary neoplasm

Table 1
Gross appearance of pancreatic lesions

very high CEA values (>800 ng/mL) are highly predictive of mucinous neoplasms (specificity >98%, but sensitivity <50%).[1] Tumor markers alone, however, cannot distinguish between benign and malignant mucinous cysts. All other markers (CA125, CA19.9, CA72-4) are increased in mucinous neoplasms and low in non-neoplastic lesions. The fluid viscosity in nonmucinous cysts is usually lower than that of serum, whereas the fluid viscosity in mucinous cysts is higher than that of serum.[17] Recent molecular studies have shown K-*ras* mutations, tumor suppressor gene mutations, and telomerase activity in neoplastic mucinous cysts.[19–21]

Several molecular studies can also be performed on pancreatic cyst fluid. One such commercially available molecular test, created by RedPath Integrated Pathology, (Pittsburgh, PA, USA), was developed specifically for pancreatic cyst fluid analysis and can also be performed on deparaffinized cell blocks. The molecular kit is called PathFinderTG and includes 3 tests[22]:

1. *K-ras* gene point mutation
2. Loss of heterozygosity (LOH) analysis using 15 preselected genomic loci associated with tumor suppressor genes
3. DNA quantity/quality measurement in cyst fluid.

Pancreatic cyst fluid showing abnormalities in 1 of these 3 molecular tests is considered abnormal and cyst fluid with high-amplitude (>75% of total DNA content) *K-ras* or LOH mutations is considered malignant.[22] The PathFinderTG test, however, is still not widely used today.

REPORTING TERMINOLOGY IN PANCREATIC CYTOPATHOLOGY

Six diagnostic categories should be used in the reporting of pancreatic FNAB: nondiagnostic, negative for malignant cells, atypical cells present, suspicious for malignancy, positive for malignant cells, and neoplastic cells present. The "nondiagnostic" category should be used when the amount of material collected is unsatisfactory because of low cellularity or when the material present does not correspond to or represent the site or lesion that was allegedly biopsied. The "negative for malignant cells" category should be used when the aspirated material consists of benign pancreatic epithelium or shows changes such as acute or chronic pancreatitis. The category "atypical cells present" should be used when cells (epithelial or mesenchymal) show atypical changes usually in the form of mild atypia and in a background of inflammation. Such changes are commonly seen in chronic pancreatitis. The "suspicious for malignancy" category should be used when atypical cells are present that are very worrisome for malignancy but are either qualitatively or quantitatively insufficient for a definite diagnosis of malignancy. Indeterminate diagnoses such as "atypical or suspicious cells present" are a result of several factors, including low specimen cellularity, gastrointestinal (GI) tract contaminants, inflammation with reactive ductal cells, poor cell preservation, and underdiagnosis.[23] The category "positive for malignant cells" should be used when cells show obvious malignant features. The "neoplastic cells present" category deserves special mention, as it encompasses situations in which cells that are present are clearly neoplastic but not clearly benign or malignant. Examples of this category include mucinous lesions (where one is unable to distinguish between a mucinous cystic neoplasm and an intraductal papillary mucinous neoplasm), solid pseudo-papillary neoplasm (a low-grade malignant neoplasm, which often behaves in a benign fashion), and pancreatic endocrine neoplasm (whose metastatic potential is unknown at the time of cytologic diagnosis).

Key Points
REPORTING TERMINOLOGY IN PANCREATIC CYTOPATHOLOGY

- Nondiagnostic

- Negative for malignant cells

- Atypical cells present

- Suspicious for malignancy

- Positive for malignant cells

- Neoplastic cells present

CONTAMINANTS IN PANCREATIC CYTOPATHOLOGY

By the very nature of the sampling technique, EUS-FNAB introduces GI contaminants into a smear.[1,5,6] This is a potential diagnostic pitfall for pathologists, as separation of gastric and duodenal contaminants from pancreatic ductal adenocarcinoma can be especially challenging. GI tract contaminants include gastric epithelium, duodenal epithelium, and GI tract mucin. Such contaminants would not be seen in a percutaneous pancreatic FNAB. Duodenal epithelium forms large, flat, or folded honeycomb sheets of evenly spaced bland epithelial cells studded by benign goblet cells (**Fig. 1**).[24] Examination of the edge of these tissue fragments will also show a distinct brush border,[1,5,24] distinguishing duodenal cells from a well-differentiated ductal carcinoma or gastric foveolar epithelium. Features favoring carcinoma over GI tract contaminants include architectural crowding, high nuclear to cytoplasmic ratio, nuclear contour irregularity, and prominent nucleoli, which would not be seen in duodenal or gastric epithelium. The immunohistochemical stain B72.3 shows some promise in being able to separate GI contaminants from pancreatic adenocarcinoma, as it shows fine perinuclear punctuate staining in gastric and duodenal epithelium, strong diffuse cytoplasmic staining in

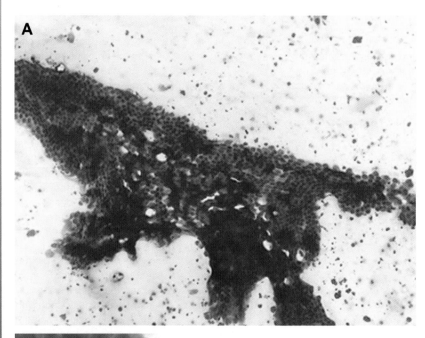

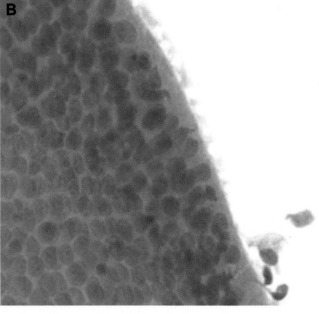

Fig. 1. (*A*) Large folded sheet of duodenal epithelial cells with interspersed goblet cells (Diff-Quik stain, ×200 magnification). (*B*) Duodenal epithelium forming sheets of evenly spaced bland cells with an indistinct peripheral brush border (Diff-Quik stain, ×400 magnification).

Differential Diagnosis and Key Points

ΔΔ CONTAMINANTS IN PANCREATIC CYTOPATHOLOGY

- Gastric epithelium may be mistaken for a mucinous neoplasm.

- Presence of monolayer sheets with mucin cups in the superficial one-third of the cell favors gastric epithelium over a mucinous neoplasm.

- Duodenal epithelium may be mistaken for a mucinous neoplasm.

- Presence of a distinct brush border and isolated goblet cells within monolayer sheets favors duodenal epithelium versus a pure population of mucin-filled cells, which favors a mucinous neoplasm.

- Mucin in the background may be a sign of a mucinous neoplasm.

- However, GI tract mucin is usually scant, thin, and streaming, as opposed to the mucin in a mucinous neoplasm, which is abundant, thick, and colloidlike.

Abbreviation: GI, gastrointestinal.

ductal adenocarcinoma, and negative staining in benign ductal epithelium.[25] The presence of isolated goblet cells (see **Fig. 1**) should also help to distinguish duodenal epithelium from a mucinous neoplasm, which would show a pure population of mucin-filled cells instead of isolated goblet cells. Gastric foveolar epithelium is even more challenging in its distinction from the epithelial cells of a mucinous neoplasm. Gastric foveolar-type epithelium is usually dispersed as monolayer sheets with cytoplasmic mucin confined to the superficial one-third of the cell's surface, forming distinct mucin cups and lacking a brush border.[5] The mucin does not fill the entire cytoplasmic compartment nor does it displace the nucleus peripherally, as it would in a mucinous neoplasm (**Fig. 2**). An intraductal papillary mucinous neoplasm may be especially difficult to differentiate from benign gastric and duodenal epithelium, especially when it shows intestinal- or gastric-type epithelial lining. GI tract mucin may also be seen in an EUS-FNAB but is usually scant, thin, and streaming in quality, unlike the more abundant, thick, colloidlike mucin seen in a mucinous neoplasm.[24] If tumor cells are

admixed with this thick mucin, this should help with the distinction from gastric epithelium.

NORMAL PANCREATIC CYTOLOGY

It is important to be familiar with normal pancreatic cytomorphology to avoid misdiagnosing these cells as malignant. Normal pancreatic cells include exocrine (acinar and ductal cells) and endocrine cells.[1,6] Pancreatic acinar cells are arranged as small, rounded groups or acini with inconspicuous lumens. Architecture is paramount to the recognition of these cells, as they typically form grapelike structures on smear (**Fig. 3**). Rare single acinar cells may also be seen and are bland with low nuclear to cytoplasmic ratio, abundant granular cytoplasm, and peripheral nuclei with fine chromatin and inconspicuous nucleoli. Pancreatic ductal cells form monolayer sheets of evenly spaced cells with well-defined cell borders, round nuclei, inconspicuous nucleoli, and fine chromatin (see **Fig. 3**). Islet cells are only rarely identified in pancreatic cytology because they are few in number and are not distinctive.

DIAGNOSIS OF PANCREATIC LESIONS

The cytologic diagnosis of pancreatic lesions is challenging and depends not only on cytomorphologic assessment, but also on clinical findings, including patient age, sex, tumor location (head, body, or tail), and gross configuration (solid, cystic, or intraductal). The most common pancreatic lesions that are sampled by FNAB are listed in **Table 2** and are discussed separately.

Key Points

NORMAL PANCREATIC CYTOPATHOLOGY

- Acinar cells are arranged singly or as grape-like clusters or acini with inconspicuous lumens.

- Cells have eccentric nuclei, fine chromatin, abundant granular cytoplasm, and inconspicuous nucleoli.

- Pancreatic ductal cells form monolayer sheets with even distribution and well-defined cell borders.

- Cells have round nuclei, inconspicuous nucleoli, and fine chromatin.

- Islet cells are only rarely seen in smears and are few in number.

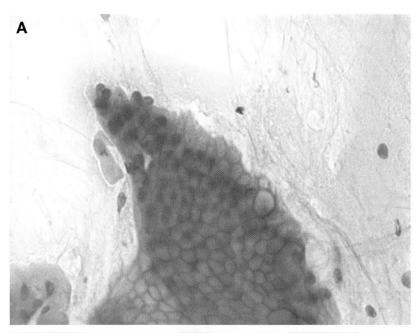

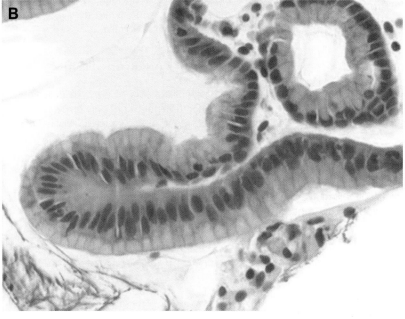

Fig. 2. Sheet (*A*) and strip (*B*) of gastric foveolar epithelium with distinct U-shaped cytoplasmic mucin cups occupying the superficial one-third of the cell surface (hematoxylin-eosin stain, ×400 magnification).

Fig. 3. (*A*) Pancreatic acinar cells arranged in rounded groups or acini with inconspicuous lumens (hematoxylin-eosin stain, ×400 magnification). (*B*) Flat monolayer honeycomb sheet of pancreatic ductal cells (hematoxylin-eosin stain, ×400 magnification).

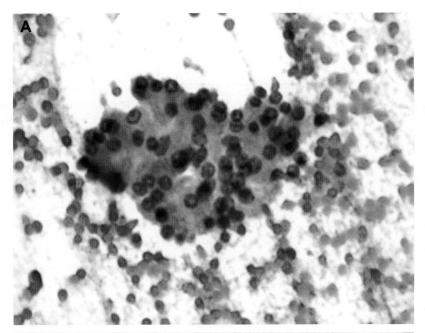

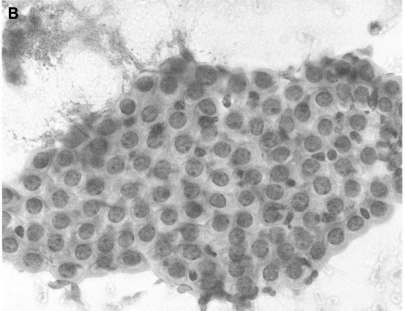

Table 2
Classification of pancreatic epithelial neoplasms

Diagnosis	%
Ductal adenocarcinoma	85
Pancreatic endocrine neoplasm	3–4
Intraductal papillary mucinous neoplasm	3–5
Mucinous cystic neoplasm	1–2
Serous cystadenoma	1–2
Solid-pseudopapillary neoplasm	1–2
Acinar cell carcinoma	1–2
Pancreatoblastoma	<1

SOLID LESIONS OF THE PANCREAS

DUCTAL ADENOCARCINOMA

Ductal adenocarcinoma is the most commonly encountered pancreatic neoplasm and accounts for 85% of all pancreatic lesions.[26] Most of these are solid, and 60% to 70% occur in the head of the pancreas of individuals between 60 and 80 years old. Tumors range from well differentiated to moderately differentiated to poorly differentiated. Poorly differentiated ductal adenocarcinoma is not usually a diagnostic challenge cytologically, as one encounters hyperchromatic, crowded groups, and single tumor cells, with fourfold anisonucleosis,[1,5] irregular nuclear contours,[27] high nuclear to cytoplasmic ratios, and macronucleoli,[6] all in a background of necrosis (**Fig. 4**). Smears are often hypercellular with 3-dimensional clusters and scattered single cells.[4] The distinction of a well-differentiated or moderately differentiated ductal adenocarcinoma from benign ductal cells is the most challenging cytologically.[5] In a well-differentiated to moderately differentiated ductal adenocarcinoma, the tumor cells form small, 3-dimensional clusters and disarrayed cohesive sheets similar to those seen in normal ductal cells (**Fig. 5**).[1,5,6] Nuclear enlargement is mild and anisonucleosis is not pronounced. Normal pancreatic acini and endocrine cells should be rare to absent in such smears. What also helps to distinguish such tumors from benign ductal cells is the slight crowding or disorder of the ductal cells (so-called "drunken honeycomb" sheets) and the slight nuclear contour irregularity (see **Fig. 5**), which are not seen in benign ductal cells.[1,5,6] The presence of mitoses does not support a diagnosis of carcinoma, as increased mitoses can be seen in chronic pancreatitis.

Sometimes cytomorphology alone is unable to distinguish such well-differentiated tumors from

Key Points
DUCTAL ADENOCARCINOMA

- Well-differentiated to moderately differentiated tumors have disarrayed cohesive sheets similar to those seen in normal ductal cells.
  - However, nuclear enlargement is mild and anisonucleosis is not pronounced.
  - Tumor cells are slightly crowded or disorderly forming "drunken honeycomb" sheets.
- Poorly differentiated tumors have crowded grouped malignant cells with hyperchromatic nuclei, fourfold anisonucleosis, irregular nuclei, macronucleoli, and high nuclear to cytoplasmic ratio, as well as single tumor cells.

△△ **Differential Diagnosis**
OF **DUCTAL ADENOCARCINOMA**

- 1- Chronic pancreatitis
  - Fourfold anisonucleosis, macronucleoli, coarse clumped chromatin, and irregular nuclear contours favor ductal adenocarcinoma over chronic pancreatitis.
  - Ductal adenocarcinoma is negative for the SMAD4 immunostain, positive for p53, and negative or weakly positive for CDX-2.
  - Reactive ductal cells are positive for SMAD4 and negative for p53 and CDX-2.
- 2- GI epithelial contaminant
  - GI epithelial contaminants are positive for CDX-2 and SMAD4 but negative for p53.

Abbreviations: CDX-2, caudal-related homeobox 2; GI, gastrointestinal; SMAD4, mothers against decapentaplegic homolog 4.

Fig. 4. Poorly differentiated ductal adenocarcinoma composed of a 3-dimensional group of neoplastic cells with (*A*) fourfold anisonucleosis, hyperchromasia, and (*B*) nuclear contour irregularity (Papanicolaou stain, ×400 magnification).

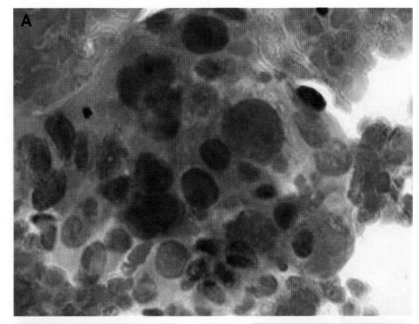

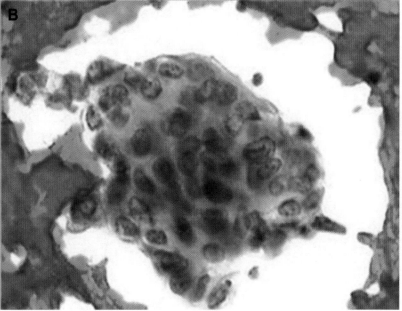

chronic pancreatitis and normal intestinal epithelium. In such situations, the most judicious practice is to report such cases as "atypical cells present" or "suspicious cells present" with a comment raising the possibility of, but not committing to, a diagnosis of malignancy. Immunohistochemical stains can also be helpful in identifying ductal adenocarcinoma. SMAD4 (mothers against decapentaplegic homolog 4)/DPC4 (deleted in pancreatic cancer, locus 4), p53, and CDX-2 (caudal-related homeobox 2) are useful in the diagnosis and distinction of ductal adenocarcinoma from chronic pancreatitis and GI epithelial contaminants.[28,29] Loss of SMAD4 expression, p53 expression, and weak or absent CDX-2 expression are typical of ductal adenocarcinoma. The atypical ductal cells of chronic pancreatitis are positive for SMAD4 and negative for p53 and

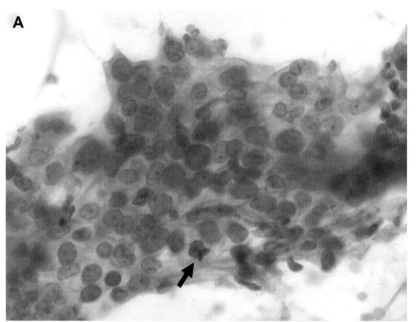

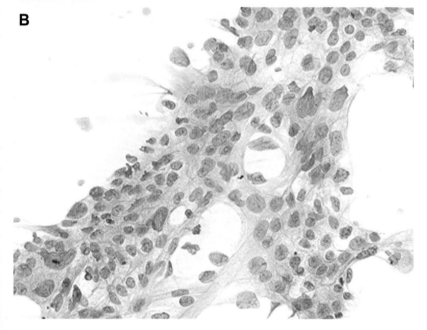

Fig. 5. (*A*) Well-differentiated ductal carcinoma composed of "drunken honeycomb" sheet of cells with slight nuclear pleomorphism, nuclear contour irregularity, and occasional abnormal mitosis (*arrow*) (Papanicolaou stain, ×400 magnification). (*B*) Moderately differentiated ductal adenocarcinoma with preserved sheetlike arrangement of cells showing nuclear crowding, moderate anisonucleosis, hyperchromasia, and nuclear contour irregularity (Papanicolaou stain, ×200 magnification).

CDX-2. GI epithelial contaminants strongly express SMAD4 and CDX-2 but are negative for p53.[28] In a study by van Heek and colleagues,[29] using a panel of K-*ras* mutation, loss of DPC4, and expression of p53, it was shown that 67% of cytologically diagnosed ductal adenocarcinomas had at least 1 of these 3 molecular alterations.

Several less common subtypes of ductal adenocarcinoma of the pancreas have been described in the cytology literature. These include adenosquamous[30,31] and undifferentiated carcinoma with osteoclastlike giant cells.[32] Adenosquamous carcinomas frequently have cellular smears with an obvious squamous population showing prominent keratinization as well as intracellular mucin and/or honeycomb glandular sheets.[30] The diagnosis of adenosquamous carcinoma is not a challenge when both components are well represented, but when the squamous component is limited, the tumor may not be readily recognized as an adenosquamous carcinoma. Adenosquamous carcinomas must also be distinguished from pure squamous cell carcinoma of the pancreas, which is extremely rare but has been reported on EUS-FNAB **(Fig. 6)**.[33] Such cases of pure squamous cell carcinoma usually represent metastases rather than true primary pancreatic tumors; therefore, correlation with clinical information is paramount to the accurate diagnosis of these cases. Pulmonary squamous cell carcinoma has been reported to metastasize to the pancreas, where it has been aspirated and diagnosed by FNAB.[34] Undifferentiated carcinoma with osteoclastlike giant cells shows an admixture of anaplastic ductal epithelium as well as benign-appearing osteoclastlike multinucleated giant cells and background mononuclear cells with variable

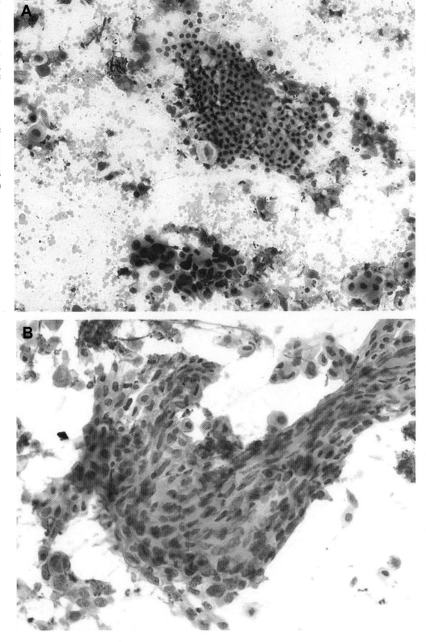

Fig. 6. Primary squamous cell carcinoma of the pancreas. (*A*) Clusters and singly dispersed malignant squamous cells are admixed with keratinous debris and a sheet of benign pancreatic ductal cells (Diff-Quik stain, ×100 magnification). (*B*) High-power view of malignant keratinized squamous cells arranged both singly and in clusters (Papanicolaou stain, ×200 magnification).

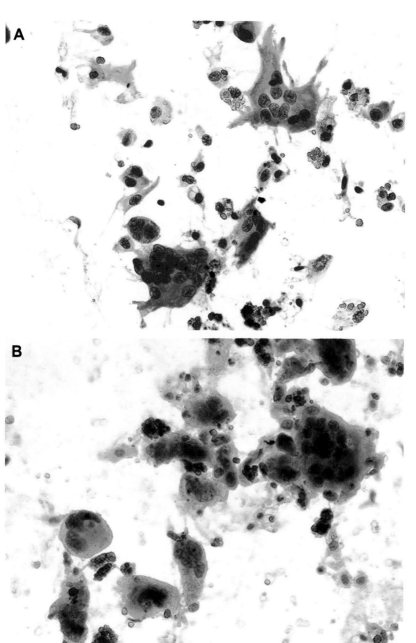

Fig. 7. (*A*) Undifferentiated carcinoma with osteoclastlike giant cells showing a mixture of anaplastic ductal epithelial cells as well as benign-appearing osteoclastlike giant cells (Papanicolaou stain, ×400 magnification). (*B*) Note benign osteoclastlike giant cells, malignant giant cells and background necrotic debris (Papanicolaou stain, ×400 magnification).

atypia ranging from bland to highly pleomorphic (**Fig. 7**).[32]

CHRONIC PANCREATITIS

Chronic pancreatitis can also present as a solid mass in the head of the pancreas. The periphery of such lesions may appear highly irregular and infiltrative, thus making it difficult to distinguish radiologically from carcinoma.[1] Cytologic specimens of chronic pancreatitis are usually of low cellularity and typically show a mixed lympho-histiocytic infiltrate, fat necrosis, and stromal fragments (**Fig. 8**).[1,5,6] The presence of reactive ductal cells in the smear background may cause cytologic confusion with ductal adenocarcinoma. Reactive ductal cells show nuclear enlargement, loss of monolayer sheets, mild to moderate nuclear crowding, and prominent nucleoli (**Fig. 9**). In contrast to adenocarcinoma, however, there is no anisonucleosis or nuclear contour irregularity in chronic pancreatitis, nor are there isolated atypical cells. Nonetheless, the accurate distinction between chronic pancreatitis and ductal adenocarcinoma requires careful correlation of radiographic, clinical, and cytologic findings. In some situations, resolution of especially challenging cases may require the use of immunohistochemistry. The atypical ductal cells in chronic pancreatitis are positive for SMAD4 and negative for p53, whereas ductal adenocarcinoma is negative for SMAD4 and positive for p53.[1,28]

Acute pancreatitis is rarely sampled by EUS-FNAB (see **Fig. 8**), as it is usually a clinical diagnosis made by correlation of presenting symptoms, imaging modalities, and laboratory tests.

PANCREATIC ENDOCRINE NEOPLASMS

Pancreatic endocrine neoplasms (PEN) account for only 3% to 4% of pancreatic neoplasms[26] and are usually solid tumors that are small in size (1 cm to 5 cm). Most arise in adults (40 to 60 years old) but can be seen at any age, although they are rare in children.[1,5] They are typically solid and are only rarely cystic. Tumors range from well differentiated to poorly differentiated. The most common type of PEN is the well-differentiated type, characterized by highly cellular smears with singly dispersed, uniform epithelial cells (**Fig. 10**). Clusters are rarely seen and are only loosely formed. Rosettelike structures may also rarely be seen (see **Fig. 10**).[35,36] Cells are round to oval and bland with eccentric nuclei containing "salt-n-pepper" chromatin and nucleoli that are usually indistinct but may occasionally be prominent (see **Fig. 10**). Cytoplasm is finely granular to oncocytic and cells are sometimes plasmacytoid in appearance because of their peripherally placed nuclei (see **Fig. 10**).[1,5,6,35] Such well-differentiated tumors can be distinguished not only by their cytomorphology but also by their immunohistochemical staining with the neuroendocrine markers (synaptophysin, chromogranin, CD56,

Key Points
PANCREATIC ENDOCRINE NEOPLASM

- Well-differentiated endocrine neoplasms have singly dispersed, uniform epithelial cells.

- Cells have eccentric nuclei, granular cytoplasm, appear plasmacytoid, contain "salt-n-pepper" chromatin, and have indistinct nucleoli.

- Cells stain positively for neuroendocrine markers such as synaptophysin, chromogranin, CD56, and CD57.

- Poorly differentiated endocrine neoplasms are rare and include small-cell carcinoma and large-cell neuroendocrine carcinoma.

- Large-cell neuroendocrine carcinoma demonstrates tumor necrosis, mitoses, and anisonucleosis, and may also have prominent nucleoli.

- Small-cell carcinoma shows small to intermediate cells with nuclear molding, "salt-n-pepper" chromatin, and crush artifact.

Key Points
CHRONIC PANCREATITIS

- May present as solid mass in pancreatic head.

- Smear shows low cellularity with mixed lymphohistiocytic infiltrate, fat necrosis, and stromal fragments.

- Reactive ductal cells may be seen in the smear background.

- Reactive ductal cells may show nuclear enlargement, loss of monolayer sheets, nuclear crowding, and prominent nucleoli resembling ductal adenocarcinoma.

- However, reactive ductal cells lack anisonucleosis or nuclear contour irregularity and isolated atypical cells are not seen.

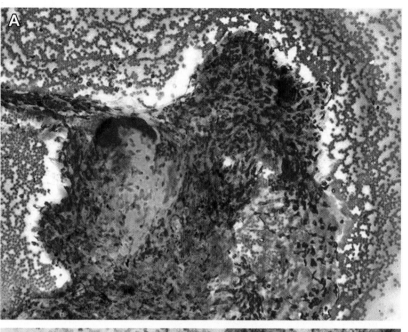

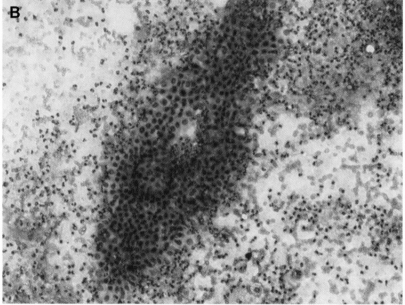

Fig. 8. (*A*) Chronic pancreatitis with pancreatic parenchyma and stromal fragments infiltrated by lymphocytes (Diff-Quik stain, ×200 magnification). (*B*) Acute pancreatitis with sheet of enlarged ductal cells admixed with abundant neutrophils and necrotic debris (Diff-Quik stain, ×200 magnification).

Fig. 9. Sheet of reactive ductal cells composed of crowded overlapping epithelial cells with slight nuclear enlargement and prominent nucleoli (hematoxylin-eosin stain, ×400 magnification).

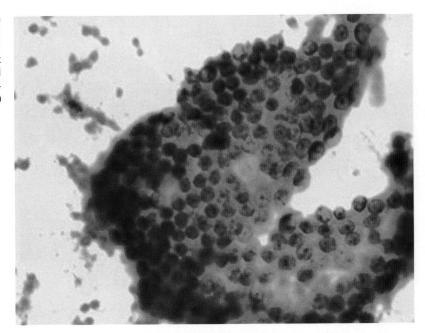

△△   ***Differential Diagnosis***
OF PANCREATIC ENDOCRINE NEOPLASM

- 1- Lymphoma
  - Also shows hypercellular smears with singly dispersed monotonous cells.
  - However, the presence of background lymphoglandular bodies favors lymphoma over PEN.
  - Tumor cells lack "salt-n-pepper" chromatin.
  - Tumor cells are positive for LCA and other lymphoid markers and negative for neuroendocrine markers.
- 2- Plasmacytoma
  - Also characterized by singly dispersed monotonous plasmacytoid cells.
  - However, tumor cells have a perinuclear hof; nuclei show "clock-face" chromatin and lack the "salt-n-pepper" chromatin.
  - Cells stain positively for CD138 and are negative for neuroendocrine markers.
- 3- Acinar cell carcinoma
  - Characterized by clusters, acinar groups and singly dispersed bland cells with abundant granular cytoplasm and prominent nucleoli.
  - Cell clusters are less common in PEN.
  - Nuclei of acinar cell carcinoma lack "salt-n-pepper" chromatin of PEN.
  - Stains positively for trypsin, chymotrypsin, and $\alpha-1-$antichymotrypsin and is negative for neuroendocrine markers.

Abbreviations: LCA, leukocyte common antigen; PEN, pancreatic endocrine neoplasm.

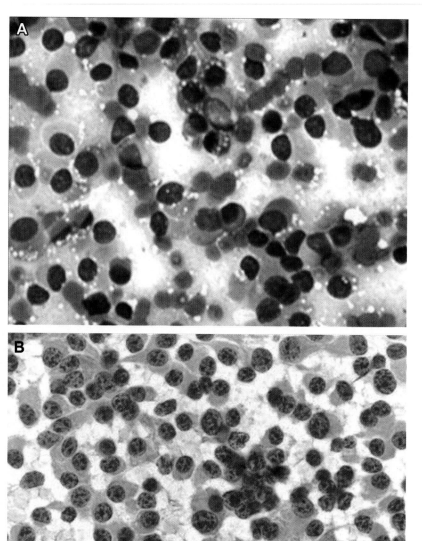

Fig. 10. Pancreatic endocrine neoplasm (well differentiated) with (*A*) hypercellular smear composed of singly dispersed, bland-appearing, uniform epithelial cells with plasmacytoid appearance (Diff-Quik stain, ×400 magnification) and (*B*) "salt-n- pepper"-type chromatin (Papanicolaou stain, ×400 magnification).

and CD57)[1,5,26,36,37] in addition to keratin (CAM5.2).[35] Poorly differentiated endocrine neoplasms are divided into small-cell carcinomas and large-cell neuroendocrine carcinomas. These are uncommon pancreatic neoplasms, which often demonstrate tumor necrosis, mitoses, anisonucleosis, and may also have large cells with prominent nucleoli.[35] Small-cell carcinoma of the pancreas resembles small-cell carcinoma of the lung and shows classical small to intermediate-

sized cells with prominent nuclear molding, "salt-n-pepper" chromatin, and prominent crush artifact (see **Fig. 10**). Large-cell neuroendocrine carcinoma resembles a poorly differentiated carcinoma that expresses neuroendocrine markers, and may also contain cytoplasmic granules that are best seen on Diff-Quik stain.

A well-differentiated PEN must be a distinguished from lymphoma, plasmacytoma, or acinar cell carcinoma. Lymphoma smears contain

Fig. 10. (*C*) Note numerous rosettes and papillary structures on cell block of well-differentiated pancreatic endocrine neoplasm (hematoxylin-eosin stain, ×100 magnification). (*D*) Small-cell carcinoma of the pancreas with small to intermediate-sized cells with high nuclear to cytoplasmic ratio and prominent nuclear molding (Diff-Quik stain, ×400 magnification).

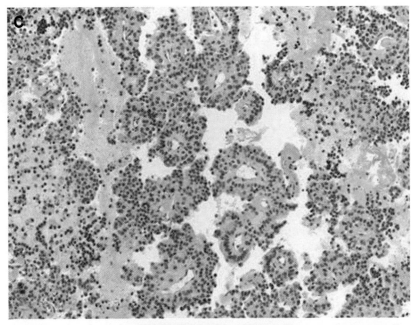

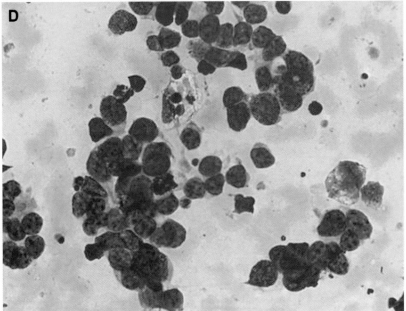

background lymphoglandular bodies, which are not seen in PEN, and lymphoma and plasmacytoma are both negative for neuroendocrine markers on immunohistochemistry.

ACINAR CELL CARCINOMA

This tumor also appears as a solid, circumscribed lesion radiographically and may be seen in the head of the pancreas. It accounts for fewer that

2% of all pancreatic exocrine tumors and tends to occur in older adults but may rarely be seen in children.[26] It is more common in men, with a Male:Female ratio of 4:1.[5] The diagnosis is especially challenging by fine-needle aspiration because of the tumor's morphologic overlap with normal pancreatic acini.[1] Smears are usually cellular with sheets, singly dispersed, and acinar groups of cells that are larger than normal acinar cells (**Fig. 11**).[38] The nuclei are also round to oval

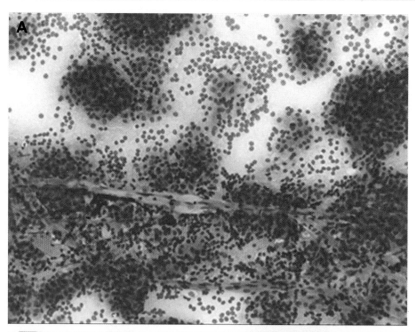

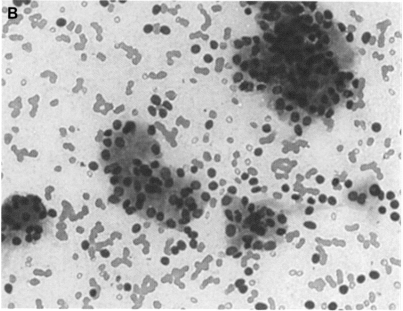

Fig. 11. Acinar cell carcinoma with (*A*) hypercellular smear composed of loose clusters and singly dispersed cells (Diff-Quik stain, ×100 magnification). (*B*) Tumor cells form loose acinar structures focally (Diff-Quik stain, ×200 magnification).

Fig. 11. (C) Acinar cells appear bland and have abundant granular cytoplasm (Diff-Quik stain, ×400 magnification). (D) Acinar cells form loose sheets of tumor cells with round to oval nuclei, fine to coarse chromatin, and single prominent nucleoli (Papanicolaou stain, ×200 magnification).

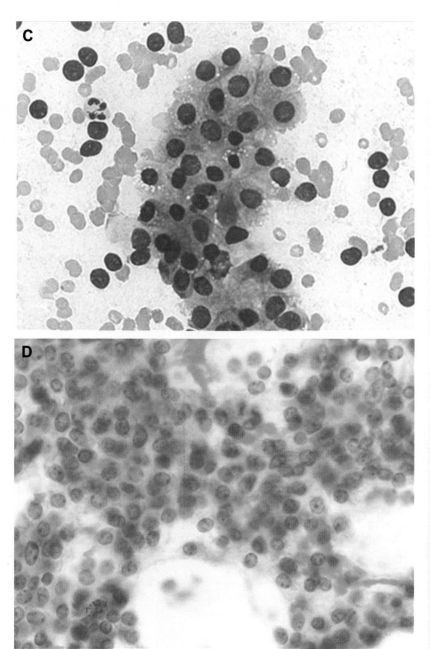

Key Points
ACINAR CELL CARCINOMA

- Solid, circumscribed lesion seen most commonly in the head of the pancreas.

- Tumor cells are arranged in sheets, acinar groups, and singly dispersed cells.

- Tumor cells are larger than normal acinar cells.

- Nuclei are round to oval and extrinsically placed with smooth contours, fine to coarse chromatin, and a single prominent nucleolus.

- Stains positively for trypsin, chymotrypsin, α-1-antichymotrypsin, and lipase.

Pitfalls
ACINAR CELL CARCINOMA

! Cytologic diagnosis is challenging because of the tumor's resemblance to normal pancreatic acini.

! Requires immunohistochemical stains for confirmation.

and the plasmacytoid cells typical of PEN are rarely seen in acinar cell carcinoma.

SOLID-PSEUDOPAPILLARY NEOPLASM

Solid-pseudopapillary neoplasm (SPN) is a low-grade malignancy that is typically large, well circumscribed, and solid, but may have a cystic component owing to secondary degeneration. These tumors are relatively rare, accounting for fewer than 3% of all pancreatic malignancies[26] and typically arise in the tail of the pancreas.[5] Tumors arise almost exclusively in women (F:M = 9:1) and usually in the third decade or adolescence, although there can be a wide age range. The cytologic features of SPN are so distinctive that accurate FNAB diagnosis can often be made before resection.[39,40] On cytology, tumors tend to result in hypercellular smears and are composed of small, uniform bland cells with

and extrinsically placed with smooth contours, fine to coarse chromatin, and a single prominent (sometimes cherry red) nucleolus (see **Fig. 11**; **Fig. 12**).[36] Periodic acid-Schiff (PAS)-positive cytoplasmic granules may be abundant.[1] Because of the fragile nature of the cells, naked nuclei are often seen and the smear background may contain granular cytoplasmic debris. Tumor cells stain positively for pancytokeratin, pancreatic enzymes trypsin, chymotrypsin, α-1-antichymotrypsin, and lipase[36] (see **Fig. 12**), as well as elastase[5] and phospholipase A2.[1] It may be challenging to distinguish acinar cell carcinoma from PEN, as both may have similar-sized discohesive cells.[36] Immunohistochemistry, however, is very helpful in distinguishing the two. In addition, the cytoplasmic granules seen in acinar cell carcinoma are only rarely seen in PEN

Differential Diagnosis
OF ACINAR CELL CARCINOMA

- Pancreatic endocrine neoplasm

  o Also has singly dispersed tumor cells.

  o Tumor cells have eccentric nuclei.

  o Nuclei have characteristic "salt-n-pepper" chromatin.

  o Cytoplasm lacks granules seen in acinar cell carcinoma.

  o Positive for neuroendocrine immunohistochemical markers.

  o Negative for trypsin, chymotrypsin, α-1-antichymotrypsin, and lipase.

Key Points
SOLID-PSEUDOPAPILLARY NEOPLASM

- Typically large, well circumscribed, and solid but may have a cystic component owing to secondary degeneration.

- Tumors arise almost exclusively in women (F:M = 9:1)

- Characteristic hypercellular smears composed of small, uniform bland cells with high nuclear to cytoplasmic ratio, fine chromatin, and inconspicuous nucleoli.

- Cells are arranged in branching, papillary clusters with fibrovascular cores.

- Nuclear grooves are rarely seen but may be prominent.

- Positive for vimentin, CD10, β-catenin, neuron-specific enolase, and CD56 and are usually negative for keratin markers.

Fig. 12. (*A*) Acinar cell carcinoma showing nuclear pleomorphism and cells with a single prominent nucleolus (Papanicolaou stain, ×600 magnification). (*B*) Cell block of acinar cell carcinoma with sheets and trabeculae of neoplastic cells (hematoxylin-eosin stain, ×200 magnification), which are positive for (*C*) trypsin immunohistochemical stains.

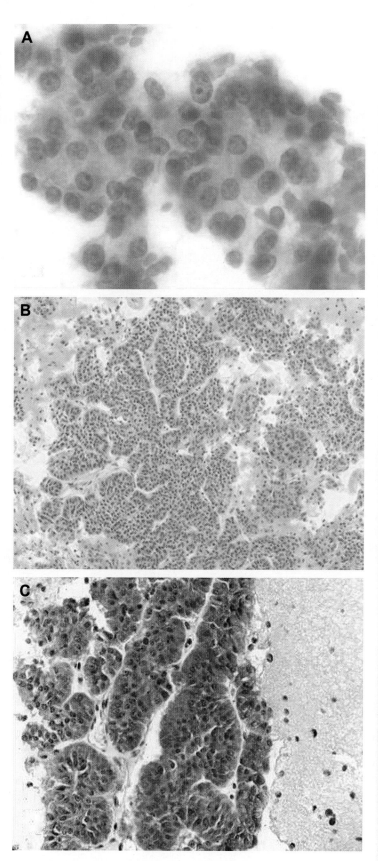

high nuclear to cytoplasmic ratio, fine chromatin, and inconspicuous nucleoli (**Fig. 13**).[6] The cells are arranged in branching, 3-layered papillary clusters, with distinct central fibrovascular cores containing myxoid-type stroma.[1,5,39] The myxoid stroma is best seen on Diff-Quik stain (see **Fig. 13**). Nuclear grooves may be rare or prominent. The smear background is either clean or hemorrhagic. The cytoplasm is typically fragile and, as a result, stripped nuclei are often seen in the smear background. Immunohistochemistry is very helpful in diagnosing these tumors, as they show characteristic positivity for vimentin, α-1-antitrypsin,[39] CD10, β-catenin, neuron-specific enolase, and CD56[1,5,26] and are usually negative for keratin markers.[6]

SPN may radiologically mimic any pancreatic tumor with a cystic component. Such tumors include serous cystadenoma, pancreatic mucinous neoplasms, and carcinomas that undergo cystic

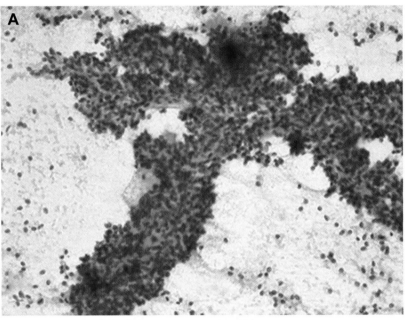

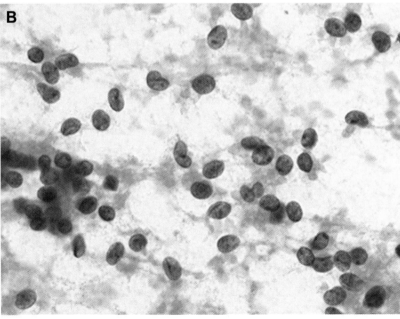

Fig. 13. (*A*) Solid-psuedopapillary neoplasm composed of hypercellular smear with branching papillary clusters (hematoxylin-eosin stain, ×200 magnification). (*B*) Numerous singly dispersed naked nuclei are present in the background, some with prominent nuclear grooves (hematoxylin-eosin stain, ×400 magnification).

Fig. 13. (*C*) The branching papillary clusters contain central myxoid-type stroma, best seen on Diff-Quik stain (×400 magnification). (*D*) Delicate papillary structure lined by small, uniform epithelial cells with high nuclear to cytoplasmic ratio, fine chromatin, and inconspicuous nucleoli (hematoxylin-eosin stain, ×400 magnification).

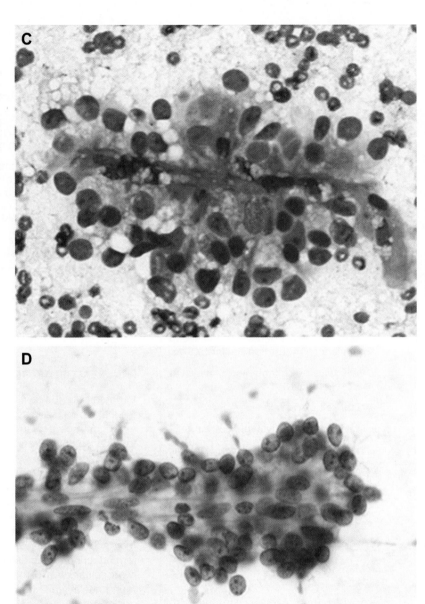

degeneration, such as acinar cell carcinoma, pancreatic endocrine neoplasm, and ductal adenocarcinoma. The cells of serous cystadenoma have clear cytoplasm and do not stain positively for CD10 and β-catenin. Mucinous neoplasms have abundant mucin in the smear background and epithelial cells with abundant cytoplasmic mucin. Acinar cell carcinoma is positive for pancreatic would not be seen in solid-pseudopapillary neoplasm.

PANCREATOBLASTOMA

Pancreatoblastomas are extremely rare malignant trilineage pancreatic neoplasms.[1,5,26] They are the most common pediatric pancreatic tumors; two-thirds arise in children, whereas one-third arise in adults.[5] Tumors are well circumscribed and often large, reaching sizes of up to 20 cm. Fifty percent of tumors occur in the head of the pancreas but they may also arise in the body or tail. Smears are typically hypercellular and because of the tumor's trilineage differentiation, they show a variety of different cell types, from (1) endocrine (resembling a PEN) to (2) exocrine (with acinar cells containing granular cytoplasm, round nuclei, and small nucleoli)[41] to (3) primitive or mesenchymal spindled cells[42] and even cartilage.[41] A distinguishing and characteristic feature of pancreatoblastoma is the presence of squamous corpuscles.[1,5,26] These however are difficult to identify on smear but can be seen on cell block.[5,41] Immunohistochemical findings in pancreatoblastoma are dependent on the tumor's line of differentiation. More than 90% of tumors are PAS-positive in the portion that shows acinar differentiation. They may also focally express neuroendocrine markers and markers of ductal differentiation (CEA and DUPAN2).

SECONDARY PANCREATIC NEOPLASMS

Various tumors may metastasize to the pancreas, causing single or multiple solid masses. These include lung (small-cell and squamous-cell

enzymes and negative for CD10 and β-catenin. Pancreatic endocrine neoplasms are positive for neuroendocrine markers and ductal adenocarcinoma shows overt malignant features, which

△△ *Differential Diagnosis* OF PANCREATOBLASTOMA

- Acinar cell carcinoma and pancreatic endocrine neoplasms

  o If exocrine component is predominant, tumor may resemble acinar cell carcinoma.

  o If endocrine component is predominant, tumor may resemble PEN.

  o Occurrence in pediatric population favors pancreatoblastoma.

  o Identification of mesenchymal elements and squamous corpuscles favor diagnosis of pancreatoblastoma.

  o Immunohistochemistry is not helpful in these cases.

Abbreviation: PEN, pancreatic endocrine neoplasm.

Key Points PANCREATIC PSEUDOCYST

- Localized collections of amylase-rich pancreatic secretions, necrotic debris, and blood.

- May have a history of alcoholism.

- Cysts are unilocular, lack septation, and most frequently occur in the tail of the pancreas.

- Cyst fluid is turbid and necrotic.

- Result in paucicellular smears with amorphous granular debris, neutrophils, macrophages, bile pigment, and fat necrosis.

- Lack true epithelial lining, but GI tract epithelial contaminants may be introduced during EUS-FNAB.

- Amylase levels are high (>250 ng/mL) and CEA levels are low.

Abbreviations: CEA, carcinoembryonic antigen; EUS-FNAB, endoscopic ultrasound-guided fine-needle aspiration biopsy; GI, gastrointestinal.

carcinoma),[1,10,34] breast, kidney,[43] and lymphoma.[6] Other less common tumors include metastases from the skin (merkel cell carcinoma),[44] ovary, colon, and stomach.[10] A history of previous malignancy is helpful in the diagnosis of these cases.

CYSTIC LESIONS OF THE PANCREAS

The primary goal of FNAB of pancreatic cystic lesions is to distinguish low-risk pancreatic cysts (serous cystadenomas, lymphoepithelial cysts, and pseudocysts) from high-risk neoplastic mucinous lesions (mucinous cystic neoplasm and intraductal papillary mucinous neoplasm). Low-risk pancreatic cysts have a low risk of harboring malignancy and are resected only when they induce symptoms or complications or when a definitive diagnosis cannot be rendered without surgical intervention. High-risk pancreatic cysts have the potential to harbor high-grade dysplasia and/or carcinoma and such lesions are usually managed surgically with partial or total pancreatectomy.

LOW-RISK PANCREATIC CYSTS

Pancreatic Pseudocysts

Pancreatic pseudocysts are localized collections of amylase-rich pancreatic secretions, necrotic debris, and blood.[5] They typically occur in the setting of acute pancreatitis (owing to postnecrotic resorption of fat necrosis). They still remain as the most common cyst occurring in the pancreas, however, they are often easily recognized by clinicians and are typically managed with conservative medical therapy, observation, or rarely by marsupialization, but are seldom resected. Therefore, surgical pathologists seldom encounter pseudocysts, unless they are removed incidentally for other pathologic conditions. The cysts are unilocular in 92% of cases,[8] lack septation, and occur most frequently in the tail of the pancreas.[5] On cytology, specimens are usually paucicellular with background amorphous granular debris, neutrophils, macrophages, yellow bile pigment, and fat necrosis (**Fig. 14**).[1,5,8] Although pseudocysts lack a true epithelial lining, GI tract epithelial contaminants may be introduced during the process of EUS-FNAB. Fibrous stroma and a variable lymphoid infiltrate, as well as normal pancreatic ducts, acini, and islet cells may also be seen.

Pancreatic pseudocysts may radiologically resemble serous cystadenomas, lymphoepithelial cysts, and pancreatic mucinous neoplasms. It is especially important to distinguish a pancreatic pseudocyst from a high-risk mucinous neoplasm-related cyst. The cyst fluid in pseudocysts is described as turbid and necrotic but is not mucinous or gelatinous, as it is in mucinous cysts. To exclude a mucinous lesion, the fluid can be stained with mucicarmine and Alcian blue (pH

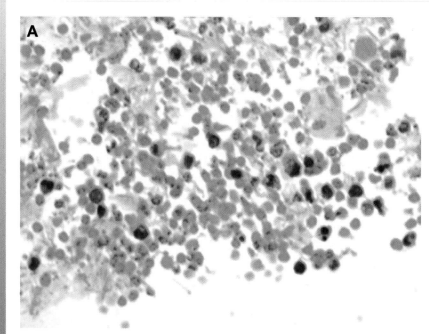

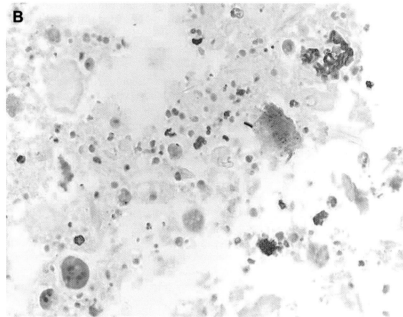

Fig. 14. Cell block sections of (*A* and *B*) pancreatic pseudocyst showing mixed inflammatory cells, blood, and yellow bile pigment (hematoxylin-eosin stain, ×400 magnification). The corresponding smears were hypocellular.

Differential Diagnosis
OF PANCREATIC PSEUDOCYST

- Other cystic pancreatic lesions

  - 1- Serous cystadenoma

    - Cyst fluid is clear in color and not turbid, as in pseudocyst.

    - Aspirates have low cellularity.

    - Smears contain low cuboidal epithelial cells with low nuclear to cytoplasmic ratio, round to oval nuclei, and inconspicuous nucleoli.

    - Cells have clear or gray-blue cytoplasm with wispy borders.

    - Lack amorphous debris, inflammatory cells, bile pigment, and fat necrosis seen in pseudocyst.

  - 2- Lymphoepithelial cyst

    - Cyst fluid is also turbid, as in pseudocyst.

    - Aspirates contain nucleated and anucleated squamous cells, amorphous debris, and lymphocytes.

    - Squamous cells are not seen in pseudocyst.

    - Amylase levels may or may not be increased in lymphoepithelial cyst.

  - 3- Pancreatic mucinous neoplasms

    - Aspirates contain thick gelatinous mucin, which is not seen in pseudocyst.

    - Cells contain abundant mucin, which is not seen in pseudocyst.

    - Lack amorphous debris, inflammatory cells, bile pigment, and fat necrosis seen in pseudocyst.

    - Unlike pseudocysts, CEA levels are often high (>200 ng/mL).

Abbreviation: CEA, carcinoembryonic antigen.

2.5), which are both negative in pseudocysts and positive in mucinous cystic lesions.[5] Amylase levels are increased (>250 ng/mL) in pseudocysts,[5] and this elevation is a result of the connection of the cyst with the pancreatic ductal system.[5] CEA levels are decreased in pseudocysts in comparison with mucinous cysts in which CEA levels are usually high (>200 ng/mL).

Pitfalls
PANCREATIC PSEUDOCYST

! May radiologically mimic other pancreatic lesions with cystic component, including serous cystadenoma, lymphoepithelial cyst, and pancreatic mucinous neoplasm.

! Smears are hypocellular with amorphous debris and few inflammatory cells, so cytologic diagnosis may be one of exclusion.

Lymphoepithelial Cysts

Lymphoepithelial cysts are extremely rare true benign pancreatic cysts, which represent approximately 0.5% of all pancreatic cysts.[45] They occur predominantly in men,[46] usually in their fifth to sixth decades.[45,47,48] Most cysts appear as hypoechoic uniloculated macrocystic masses in the tail and/or body of the pancreas, but they may also be multiloculated[47,48] or extra/peripancreatic.[48] They are not connected to the main pancreatic duct. On aspiration, lymphoepithelial cysts contain cells similar to those seen in their histologic counterparts. FNAB often reveals variably cellular smears composed of abundant mature nucleated and anucleated squamous cells in a background of amorphous keratinous debris (**Fig. 15**). In addition, the smear background contains a variable number of mature lymphocytes, as well

Key Points
LYMPHOEPITHELIAL CYST

- Rare, benign true pancreatic cyst (~0.5% of all pancreatic cysts).

- Cysts are uniloculated, macrocystic masses in the tail and/or body of the pancreas, but may be multiloculated or peripancreatic.

- Contain turbid fluid on aspiration.

- Smears are cellular and composed of nucleated and anucleated squamous cells, amorphous keratinous debris, lymphocytes, histiocytes, and giant cells.

- Cytologic diagnosis is relatively straightforward.

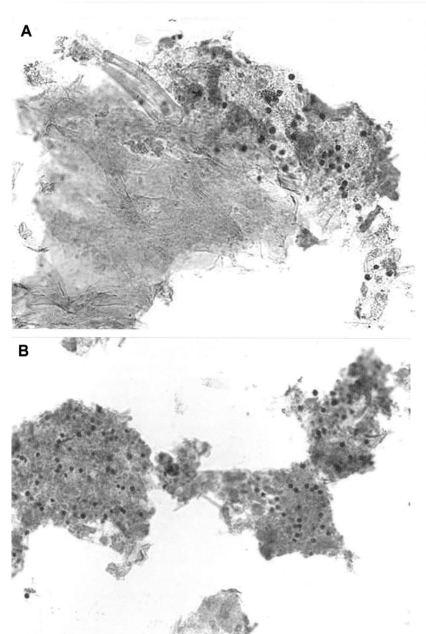

Fig. 15. Lymphoepithelial cyst composed of (*A*) a cluster of acellular squamous cells and adjacent mature lymphocytes (Papanicolaou stain, ×200 magnification). (*B*) Lymphocytes are embedded in amorphous debris (Papanicolaou stain, ×200 magnification).

as histiocytes and multinucleated foreign-body–type giant cells.[47–49] The cytologic diagnosis of lymphoepithelial cyst is relatively straightforward, and accurate diagnosis obviates the need for more radical surgical intervention and is helpful in preoperative surgical planning.

The most significant cytologic differential diagnoses of a lymphoepithelial cyst are pancreatic pseudocyst, dermoid cyst of the pancreas, mucinous pancreatic neoplasms, and primary squamous cell or adenosquamous carcinoma of the pancreas. Although the pancreatic pseudocyst also contains inflammatory cells, amorphous debris, and cholesterol crystals, a predominance of squamous cells is not a feature. Dermoid cysts, extremely rare in the pancreas,[50,51] are characterized with a mixture of squamous epithelium as well as hair follicles and other teratomatous

Fig. 15. (*C*) Cluster of keratinous debris (Papanicolaou stain, ×200 magnification). (*D*) Cell block section with benign pancreatic ductal cells, scattered lymphocytes, and laminated keratin (hematoxylin-eosin stain, ×200 magnification).

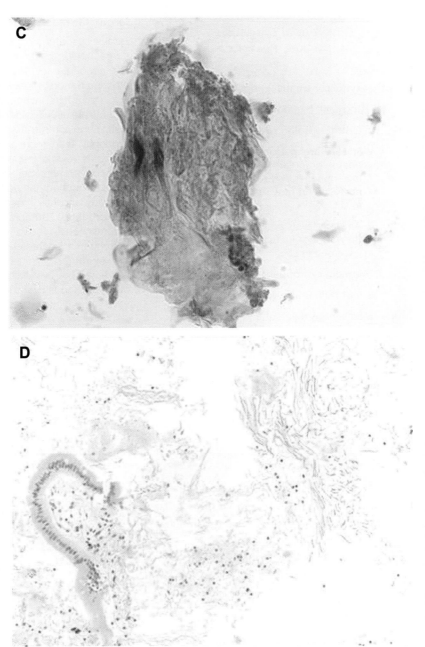

elements, such as respiratory epithelium. Mucinous pancreatic neoplasms have abundant background mucin as well as mucin-filled epithelial cells, but keratinous debris and squamous epithelium are not seen. Primary or metastatic squamous cell and adenosquamous carcinomas of the pancreas may both contain keratinous material and squamous cells, but the squamous epithelium would show obvious malignant features, including nuclear pleomorphism, hyperchromasia, prominent nucleoli, and abnormal mitoses, features that would not be seen in a lymphoepithelial cyst.

△△ **Differential Diagnosis**
OF LYMPHOEPITHELIAL CYST

- Other cystic pancreatic lesions
  - ○ 1- Pancreatic pseudocyst
    - Cyst fluid is also turbid, as in LEC.
    - Smears are paucicellular with amorphous granular debris, neutrophils, macrophages, bile pigment, and fat necrosis and lack squamous cells seen in LEC.
    - Amylase levels are increased, whereas they are not increased or only slightly increased in LEC.
  - ○ 2- Dermoid cyst of pancreas
    - Cyst fluid is also turbid, as in LEC.
    - Smears contain squamous cells similar to LEC.
    - However, hair follicles and other teratomatous elements, such as respiratory epithelium, are also present.
  - ○ 3- Pancreatic mucinous neoplasms
    - Aspirates contain thick gelatinous mucin, which is not seen in LEC.
    - Cells contain abundant mucin, which is not seen in LEC.
    - Lack squamous cells and inflammatory cells that are seen in LEC.
    - Unlike LEC, CEA levels are often high (>200 ng/mL).
  - ○ 4- Squamous cell carcinoma or adenosquamous carcinoma of pancreas
    - Both may appear cystic on radiology if they undergo degeneration.
    - Aspirates contain either pure squamous population or admixture of glandular and squamous cells.
    - Squamous cells show obvious malignant features, unlike LEC.

Abbreviations: CEA, carcinoembryonic antigen; LEC, lymphoepithelial cyst.

Serous Cystadenoma

Serous cystadenoma or microcystic adenoma is a rare benign cystic neoplasm of the pancreas that accounts for 1% to 2% of all pancreatic exocrine tumors. Most are discovered incidentally in older adults, who are often asymptomatic. Patients are usually older than those with mucinous cystic neoplasms and women are affected far more frequently than men, unlike intraductal papillary mucinous cystic neoplasms, which are more common in men. Serous cystadenomas can be found throughout the pancreas but tend to involve the body and tail.[18] Because of their multilocular nature, these tumors have a characteristic circumscribed "soap bubble" radiologic appearance, a characteristic central stellate scar, and starburst or sunburst calcifications.[52] On aspiration, the cyst fluid is usually not mucoid, as it is in mucinous cystic lesions, but is instead thin, watery, and clear in color. Aspirates have low cellularity, which often leads to their being read as "nondiagnostic" on FNAB. Smears contain a few small clusters, sheets, and single bland, low cuboidal epithelial cells with abundant clear PAS-positive cytoplasm,[18] low nuclear to cytoplasmic ratio, round to oval nuclei, and inconspicuous nucleoli (**Fig. 16**).[53] This serous epithelium is unfortunately seen only in the aspirates of fewer than 20% of cases.[18] Nuclear grooves may also rarely be seen and chromatin may appear slightly

 Key Points
SEROUS CYSTADENOMA

- Classical multilocular "soap bubble" radiologic appearance with central stellate scar and starburst calcifications.

- Aspirated fluid is thin, watery, and clear.

- Aspirates have low cellularity and contain few cuboidal epithelial cells in clusters, sheets, and singly, with abundant clear PAS-positive cytoplasm.

- Cell blocks may show fibrous stroma and variably sized cysts lined by flat-to-low, clear cuboidal cells.

- Cells are diffusely positive for keratin (AE1/AE3) and CA19.9. EMA is focally positive.

- Amylase and CEA levels are low and mucicarmine stain is negative in cells.

Abbreviations: EMA, epithelial membrane antigen; PAS, periodic acid Schiff.

Fig. 16. Serous cystadenoma with sheets and singly dispersed cuboidal and columnar cells with low nuclear to cytoplasmic ratio, pale blue cytoplasm, and bland nuclei (Papanicolaou stain, ×200 magnification [A] and ×400 magnification [B]). (*Courtesy of* Dr Reetesh Pai, Stanford University, Stanford, CA.)

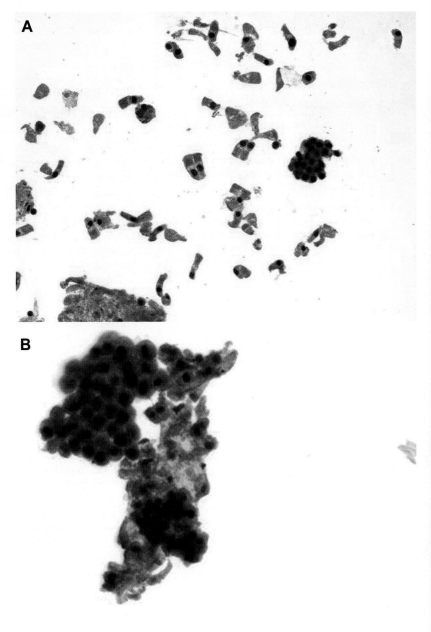

coarse in some cases.[53] The cytoplasm of epithelial cells may appear gray-blue with wispy borders on Papanicolaou stain (see **Fig. 16**). Cell blocks from aspirated tumors may show fibrous stroma and variably sized cysts lined by flat-to-low cuboidal epithelium.[53] Fibrous stroma may also be seen on smear material but is more easily identified on cell

blocks. Keratin (AE1/AE3) and CA19.9 are both diffusely and strongly positive in epithelial cells, whereas epithelial membrane antigen (EMA) is only focally positive.

The amylase and CEA levels of serous cystadenomas are low and the mucicarmine stain is negative in the cytoplasm of the epithelial cells, making

△△ *Differential Diagnosis*
OF SEROUS CYSTADENOMA

- Other cystic pancreatic lesions

  ○ 1- Pancreatic pseudocyst

    ▪ Cysts lack "soap-bubble" appearance on ultrasound.

    ▪ Unlike a serous cystadenoma's thin and clear fluid, pseudocysts contain turbid fluid on aspiration.

    ▪ Smears contain amorphous granular debris, inflammatory cells, bile pigment, and fat necrosis, whereas in serous cystadenoma there are rare epithelial cells, which appear cuboidal with clear to gray-blue PAS-positive cytoplasm.

    ▪ Amylase levels are increased.

  ○ 2- Lymphoepithelial cyst

    ▪ Unlike multiloculated serous cystadenoma, lymphoepithelial cyst is uniloculated and macrocystic.

    ▪ Contain turbid fluid on aspiration.

    ▪ Smears are composed of squamous cells, keratinous debris, and lymphocytes.

  ○ 3- Pancreatic mucinous neoplasms

    ▪ Aspirates contain thick gelatinous mucin

    ▪ Cells contain abundant mucicarmine-positive mucin, whereas serous cystadenoma has PAS-positive clear cytoplasm.

Abbreviation: PAS, periodic acid-Schiff.

distinction from pancreatic pseudocyst and mucinous neoplasms possible, respectively. Because of the absence of granular debris, inflammatory cells, and bile pigment, serous cystadenoma can be distinguished from pancreatic pseudocyst on cytology. Asymptomatic tumors have no specific surgical treatment recommendations[18]; hence, accurate cytologic diagnosis is important in preventing unnecessary surgery with its associated risks. Although adequate FNAB smears in conjunction with clinical and radiologic data are helpful in facilitating their diagnosis, some studies have shown that the accuracy of preoperative diagnosis of serous cystadenoma by imaging, cytology, and chemical analysis is as low as 20%.[18,52]

HIGH-RISK PANCREATIC CYSTS

Mucinous Pancreatic Neoplasms

There are 2 distinct primary mucin-producing neoplastic pancreatic cysts. These include mucinous cystic neoplasm (MCN) and intraductal papillary mucinous neoplasm (IPMN), together accounting for 5% of all pancreatic neoplasms.[5] These tumors are considered high risk because of their association with dysplasia and underlying carcinoma. They are hereafter described together because of their overlapping cytologic features.

The distinction between MCN and IPMN on cytology is extremely difficult,[1] and is not recommended by some.[5] There are certain findings, however, that may favor one over the other, as MCNs are distinct from IPMNs clinically, radiologically, and, to some extent, pathologically. Although most MCNs arise in the body and tail of the pancreas (with 10% arising in the pancreatic head), 70% of IPMNs arise in the head of the pancreas.[5] Most patients with MCN are women (Male:Female ratio of 1:20)[26] between the ages of 40 and 50 years,[54] whereas most patients with IPMN are older adults, older than 60, and men are slightly more frequently affected than women. MCNs are not connected to nor do they arise from the main pancreatic duct or its branches. Conversely, IPMNs are always connected to the main pancreatic duct or one of its branches as single or multiple cysts.[55,56]

On aspiration, both IPMN and MCN contain abundant thick mucin, which is difficult to draw into and express from the needle. Similarly, the background mucin is very thick and colloidlike, as opposed to the normal thin mucin that is seen in the GI tract (**Fig. 17**). Smear patterns show variable cellularity ranging from low in low-grade lesions to high in high-grade lesions.[55,57] Both tumors contain flat sheets and clusters of bland-appearing columnar cells with abundant intracytoplasmic mucin (**Figs. 18** and **19**). The mucin fills the entire cytoplasm and displaces the nucleus to the periphery or base of the cell, unlike the apical mucin cup seen in gastric foveolar epithelium. The epithelial cells in IPMN may also show gastric, pancreatobiliary, or oncocytic differentiation. MCNs have a subepithelial ovarian-type fibrous stroma, which is only rarely sampled on FNAB smears.[5] Cytologic atypia, in the form of hypercellularity, crowding, loss of polarity,

Fig. 17. Abundant thick colloidlike mucin seen in pancreatic mucinous neoplasms on (*A*) Diff-Quik stain (×200 magnification) and (*B*) Papanicolaou stain (×100 magnification).

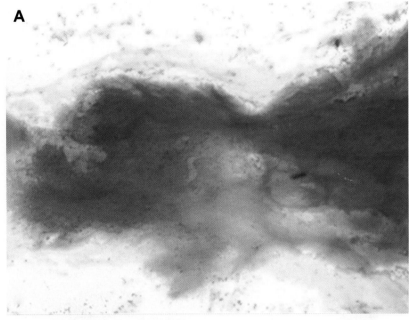

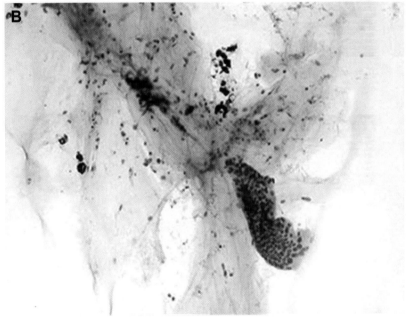

hyperchromasia, pleomorphism, high nuclear to cytoplasmic ratio, and nucleoli (see **Fig. 19**) can be seen in either tumor depending on the presence and degree of dysplasia, as well as the presence or absence of carcinoma,[54,58] but is more often seen in IPMN. Tumor cells forming elongated papillary clusters of mucinous epithelium highly favors the diagnosis of IPMN and is unusual in MCN (see **Fig. 19**).[1,5,58] IPMN with low-grade dysplasia tends to have clean backgrounds or contain less mucin and is usually paucicellular. They may be extremely difficult to differentiate from GI contaminants. The presence of a brush border and interspersed goblet cells (in duodenal

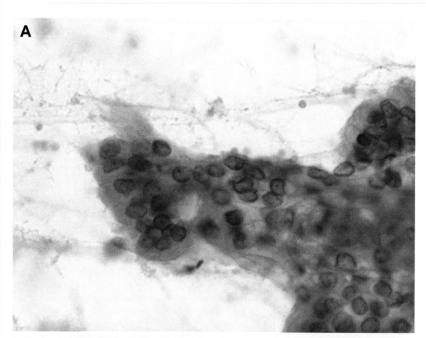

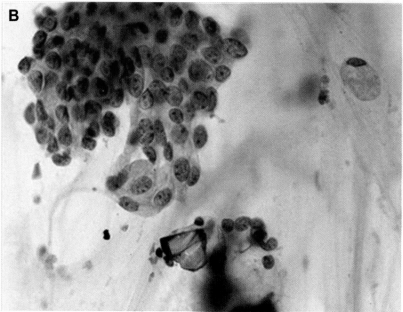

Fig. 18. Mucinous cystic neoplasm composed of (*A*) sheets of mucin-containing bland epithelial cells (hematoxylin-eosin stain, ×200 magnification). (*B*) Epithelial cells show slight nuclear atypia and hyperchromasia. Note background mucin (Papanicolaou stain, ×400 magnification). (*Courtesy of* Mary Ann Friedlander, CT [ASCP], Memorial Sloan-Kettering Cancer Center, New York, NY.)

epithelium) favors the diagnosis of GI contaminants over mucinous cysts. IPMNs with moderate to severe dysplasia have glandular fragments with nuclear crowding, loss of polarity, hyperchromasia, and high nuclear to cytoplasmic ratios (see **Fig. 19**). Necrosis and inflammation are common in IPMNs with high-grade dysplasia. The best correlate of invasion in IPMNs is the presence of necrosis[52,59]; however, this cannot be used to definitively diagnose invasion in these lesions on cytology alone.

Correlation of the cyst's location with the EUS-FNAB approach is important for accurate diagnosis of these tumors. Because MCNs arise in the body and tail of the pancreas, they are often sampled by the transgastric approach; hence, one should beware of gastric epithelial contamination.[58] Because IPMNs often arise in the head of the pancreas, they are most frequently sampled by trans-duodenal EUS-FNAB; hence, duodenal epithelial contamination is possible.[5,58]

Fig. 18. (*C*) Intracytoplasmic mucin pushes the nuclei to the periphery (*arrow*) unlike that of gastric foveolar epithelium (Papanicolaou stain, ×400 magnification). The intracellular mucin is highlighted by mucicarmine stain (*inset*) (×600 magnification). (*D*) Mucinfilled epithelial cells form clusters resembling foam cells (Diff-Quik stain, ×400 magnification).

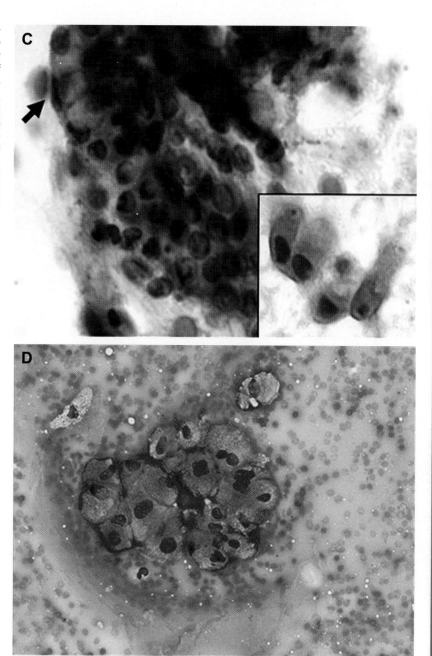

Additional tests to make the diagnosis of a pancreatic mucinous neoplasm include tumor markers. High CEA levels (>200 ng/mL) are seen in both MCN and IPMN. Amylase levels are high in IPMN[5] (because of their connection with the main pancreatic duct) and are low in MCN. Other tumor markers that are elevated in mucinous cysts include CA72.4, CA19.9,[60,61] CA125, and CA15-3.[17] These, however, are unable to distinguish between MCN and IPMN, and have also been shown to be elevated in ductal adenocarcinomas with cystic degeneration. Both MCN and IPMN show positivity for intracytoplasmic and extracytoplasmic mucin (see **Fig. 18**). Several studies

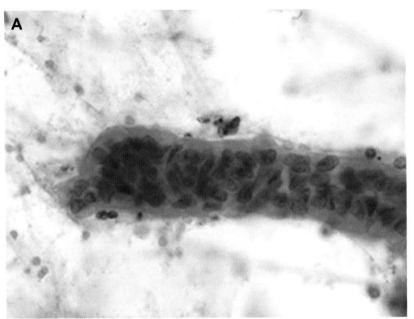

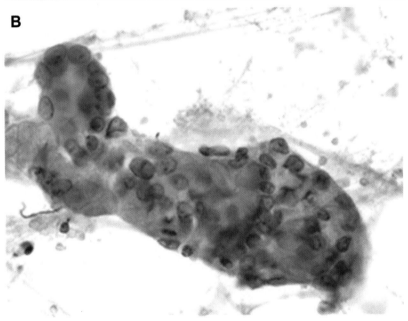

Fig. 19. Intraductal papillary mucinous neoplasm with (*A*) distinct elongated papilla lined by crowded cells with overlapping, hyperchromatic, irregular nuclei (hematoxylin-eosin stain, ×400 magnification). (*B*) Papillary cluster of cells with nuclear hyperchromasia and nuclear contour irregularity (hematoxylineosin stain, ×400 magnification).

have examined the use of B72.3 immunohistochemical stain in distinguishing GI tract contaminants from neoplastic mucinous epithelium[24,25] and have shown that GI contaminants demonstrate punctuate perinuclear staining, whereas neoplastic mucinous epithelium demonstrates diffuse cytoplasmic staining. The distinction between MCN and IPMN on cytology should be discouraged.

The best diagnosis for such mucinous lesions is "neoplastic cells present, pancreatic mucinous neoplasm."

Mucin-producing neoplastic pancreatic cysts must also be distinguished from pancreatic mucinous (colloid) adenocarcinoma. The mucinous adenocarcinoma can be distinguished from IPMN and MCN by the degree of cytologic atypia including

Key Points
MUCIN-PRODUCING NEOPLASTIC PANCREATIC CYSTS

Mucinous cystic neoplasm	Intraductal papillary mucinous neoplasm
• Most arise in body and tail of the pancreas.	• Most (70%) arise in the head of the pancreas.
• The cysts do not arise from nor are they connected to the main pancreatic duct.	• Cysts arise from the main pancreatic duct or its branches.
• Flat sheets and clusters of columnar cells with abundant intracytoplasmic mucin.	• Flat sheets and clusters of columnar cells with abundant intracytoplasmic mucin.
• Cysts have a classical subepithelial ovarian-type fibrous stroma (which is unfortunately not seen on FNAB).	• The epithelial cells in IPMN may also show pancreatobiliary or gastric differentiation. • No ovarian-type fibrous stroma.
• Spectrum of dysplasia and associated invasive carcinoma can be seen.	• Spectrum of dysplasia and associated invasive carcinoma can be seen.
• Amylase levels are often low because of the lack of connection to the pancreatic ducts.	• Amylase levels are often high because of the cyst's connection to pancreatic ducts.
• CEA levels are usually high (>200 ng/mL).	• CEA levels are usually high (>200 ng/mL).

Abbreviations: CEA, carcinoembryonic antigen; FNAB, fine-needle aspiration biopsy.

nuclear hyperchromasia, pleomorphism, increased mitoses, and necrosis, as well as signet-ring cells (**Fig. 20**). Mucin (MUC) immunohistochemistry is also helpful in diagnosing mucinous (colloid) adenocarcinoma and differentiating it from mucin-producing neoplastic cysts. Mucinous (colloid) adenocarcinoma and IPMN are both positive for MUC2 and negative for MUC1.[62] IPMNs are typically positive for MUC5AC regardless of the subtype. Most main duct IPMNs are intestinal type

△△ **Differential Diagnosis**
OF PANCREATIC MUCINOUS NEOPLASMS

• Other cystic pancreatic lesions

  ○ 1- Pancreatic pseudocyst

   ▪ Cyst fluid is turbid unlike mucinous neoplasms where it is mucoid or gelatinous.

   ▪ Smears contain amorphous granular debris, inflammatory cells, bile pigment, and fat necrosis, whereas in mucinous neoplasms there is thick colloidlike background mucin and mucin-filled mucicarmine-positive epithelial cells.

  ○ 2- Lymphoepithelial cyst

   ▪ Cysts contain turbid fluid on aspiration.

   ▪ Smears are composed of squamous cells, keratinous debris, and lymphocytes, which are not seen in mucinous neoplasms.

  ○ 3- Serous cystadenoma

   ▪ Cyst fluid is clear in color and not mucoid or gelatinous.

   ▪ Aspirates have low cellularity and contain cuboidal cells with clear cytoplasm, unlike mucinous neoplasms, which have variable cellularity and contain mucin-filled epithelial cells.

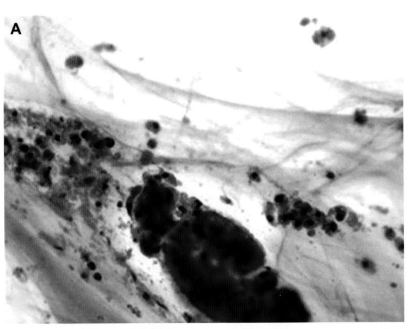

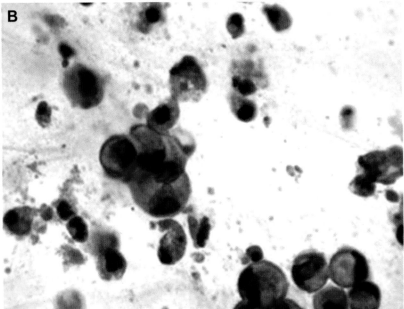

Fig. 20. Mucinous adeno-carcinoma. Note the presence of (*A*) abundant background mucin and necrotic debris, as well as (*B*) malignant cells both singly and in clusters, with rare signet-ring cells (hematoxylin-eosin stain, ×400 magnification).

and express CDX-2/MUC2 diffusely in their papillary component. Branch duct IPMNs tend to be gastric and lack MUC2/CDX-2 (with the exception of rare goblet cells) and also lack MUC1. Oncocytic IPMNs are characterized by MUC6, and pancreatobiliary IPMNs are rare and show MUC1 expression (at the luminal membranes and cytoplasm). The latter is highly similar to the newly recognized entity of intraductal tubulopapillary carcinoma (ITPN) of the pancreas, which is characterized by nonmucinous cells and prominent (or exclusive) tubular configuraton.[63–65]

> **Pitfalls**
> **PANCREATIC MUCINOUS NEOPLASMS**
>
> ! May radiologically mimic other pancreatic lesions with cystic component, including pancreatic pseudocyst, lymphoepithelial cyst, and serous cystadenoma.
>
> ! Cytologic distinction between mucinous cystic neoplasm and intraductal papillary mucinous neoplasm is often impossible and is not recommended by some.

Noninvasive MCN is MUC2-negative and MUC1-negative, whereas invasive MCN is MUC1-positive and MUC2-negative.[66]

SUMMARY

In summary, the cytologic evaluation of pancreatic lesions is a complex and challenging task, as the pancreas is the site of numerous complex cystic and solid ductal, acinar, and neuroendocrine neoplasms and cysts, each with different therapeutic and prognostic implications. However, it is a task that must be mastered because of the increasing popularity of endoscopic ultrasound-guided fine-needle aspiration biopsies. Correlation of cytology with clinical and imaging data is paramount to accurate diagnosis. The presence of a cytotechnologist or cytopathologist at the time of aspiration dramatically improves adequacy rates and ensures appropriate specimen triage with collection of material for additional studies, such as tumor markers, immunohistochemistry, and enzyme analysis. The accurate recognition of GI contaminants in endoscopically guided aspirates cannot be overstated.

REFERENCES

1. Shen J, Kindelberger DW. Pancreas and biliary tree. In: Cibas ES, Ducatman BS, editors. Cytology: diagnostic principles and clinical correlates. 3rd edition. Philadelphia: Saunders; 2009. p. 385–402.

2. Centeno BA. Fine needle aspiration biopsy of the pancreas. Clin Lab Med 1998;18(3):401–27, v–vi.

3. Ekberg O, Bergenfeldt M, Aspelin P, et al. Reliability of ultrasound-guided fine-needle biopsy of pancreatic masses. Acta Radiol 1988;29(5):535–9.

4. Bardales RH, Stelow EB, Mallery S, et al. Review of endoscopic ultrasound-guided fine-needle aspiration cytology. Diagn Cytopathol 2006;34(2):140–75.

5. Pitman MB, Deshpande V. Endoscopic ultrasound-guided fine needle aspiration cytology of the pancreas: a morphological and multimodal approach to the diagnosis of solid and cystic mass lesions. Cytopathology 2007;18(6):331–47.

6. Mitsuhashi T, Ghafari S, Chang CY, et al. Endoscopic ultrasound-guided fine needle aspiration of the pancreas: cytomorphological evaluation with emphasis on adequacy assessment, diagnostic criteria and contamination from the gastrointestinal tract. Cytopathology 2006;17(1):34–41.

7. Erickson RA, Garza AA. Impact of endoscopic ultrasound on the management and outcome of pancreatic carcinoma. Am J Gastroenterol 2000;95(9):2248–54.

8. Gonzalez Obeso E, Murphy E, Brugge W, et al. Pseudocyst of the pancreas: the role of cytology and special stains for mucin. Cancer 2009;117(2):101–7.

9. Brandt KR, Charboneau JW, Stephens DH, et al. CT- and US-guided biopsy of the pancreas. Radiology 1993;187(1):99–104.

10. David O, Green L, Reddy V, et al. Pancreatic masses: a multi-institutional study of 364 fine-needle aspiration biopsies with histopathologic correlation. Diagn Cytopathol 1998;19(6):423–7.

11. Di Stasi M, Lencioni R, Solmi L, et al. Ultrasound-guided fine needle biopsy of pancreatic masses: results of a multicenter study. Am J Gastroenterol 1998;93(8):1329–33.

12. Robins DB, Katz RL, Evans DB, et al. Fine needle aspiration of the pancreas. In quest of accuracy. Acta Cytol 1995;39(1):1–10.

13. Carrara S, Arcidiacono PG, Mezzi G, et al. Pancreatic endoscopic ultrasound-guided fine needle aspiration: complication rate and clinical course in a single centre. Dig Liver Dis 2010;42(7):520–3.

14. Levin DP, Bret PM. Percutaneous fine-needle aspiration biopsy of the pancreas resulting in death. Gastrointest Radiol 1991;16(1):67–9.

15. Bergenfeldt M, Genell S, Lindholm K, et al. Needle-tract seeding after percutaneous fine-needle biopsy of pancreatic carcinoma. Case report. Acta Chir Scand 1988;154(1):77–9.

16. Bellizzi AM, Stelow EB. Pancreatic cytopathology: a practical approach and review. Arch Pathol Lab Med 2009;133(3):388–404.

17. Lewandrowski KB, Southern JF, Pins MR, et al. Cyst fluid analysis in the differential diagnosis of pancreatic cysts. A comparison of pseudocysts, serous cystadenomas, mucinous cystic neoplasms, and mucinous cystadenocarcinoma. Ann Surg 1993;217(1):41–7.

18. Belsley NA, Pitman MB, Lauwers GY, et al. Serous cystadenoma of the pancreas: limitations and pitfalls of endoscopic ultrasound-guided fine-needle aspiration biopsy. Cancer 2008;114(2):102–10.

19. Khalid A, McGrath KM, Zahid M, et al. The role of pancreatic cyst fluid molecular analysis in predicting cyst pathology. Clin Gastroenterol Hepatol 2005;3(10):967–73.

20. Schoedel KE, Finkelstein SD, Ohori NP. K-Ras and microsatellite marker analysis of fine-needle aspirates from intraductal papillary mucinous neoplasms of the pancreas. Diagn Cytopathol 2006;34(9): 605–8.

21. Zhou GX, Huang JF, Li ZS, et al. Detection of K-ras point mutation and telomerase activity during endoscopic retrograde cholangiopancreatography in diagnosis of pancreatic cancer. World J Gastroenterol 2004;10(9):1337–40.

22. Shen J, Brugge WR, Dimaio CJ, et al. Molecular analysis of pancreatic cyst fluid: a comparative analysis with current practice of diagnosis. Cancer 2009; 117(3):217–27.

23. Payne M, Staerkel G, Gong Y. Indeterminate diagnosis in fine-needle aspiration of the pancreas: reasons and clinical implications. Diagn Cytopathol 2009;37(1):21–9.

24. Nagle JA, Wilbur DC, Pitman MB. Cytomorphology of gastric and duodenal epithelium and reactivity to B72.3: a baseline for comparison to pancreatic lesions aspirated by EUS-FNAB. Diagn Cytopathol 2005;33(6):381–6.

25. Nawgiri RS, Nagle JA, Wilbur DC, et al. Cytomorphology and B72.3 labeling of benign and malignant ductal epithelium in pancreatic lesions compared to gastrointestinal epithelium. Diagn Cytopathol 2007; 35(5):300–5.

26. Klimstra DS, Pitman MB, Hruban RH. An algorithmic approach to the diagnosis of pancreatic neoplasms. Arch Pathol Lab Med 2009;133(3):454–64.

27. Cohen MB, Egerter DP, Holly EA, et al. Pancreatic adenocarcinoma: regression analysis to identify improved cytologic criteria. Diagn Cytopathol 1991;7(4):341–5.

28. Shen J, Cibas ES, Qian X. The immunohistochemical expression pattern of SMAD4, p53 and CDX-2 is helpful in diagnosing pancreatic adenocarcinoma in endoscopic ultrasound-guided fine needle aspiration (EUS-FNA). Mod Pathol 2007;20(Suppl 2):83A.

29. van Heek T, Rader AE, Offerhaus GJ, et al. K-ras, p53, and DPC4 (MAD4) alterations in fine-needle aspirates of the pancreas: a molecular panel correlates with and supplements cytologic diagnosis. Am J Clin Pathol 2002;117(5):755–65.

30. Rahemtullah A, Misdraji J, Pitman MB. Adenosquamous carcinoma of the pancreas: cytologic features in 14 cases. Cancer 2003;99(6):372–8.

31. Wilczynski SP, Valente PT, Atkinson BF. Cytodiagnosis of adenosquamous carcinoma of the pancreas. Use of intraoperative fine needle aspiration. Acta Cytol 1984;28(6):733–6.

32. Layfield LJ, Bentz J. Giant-cell containing neoplasms of the pancreas: an aspiration cytology study. Diagn Cytopathol 2008;36(4):238–44.

33. Lai LH, Romagnuolo J, Adams D, et al. Primary squamous cell carcinoma of pancreas diagnosed by EUS-FNA: a case report. World J Gastroenterol 2009;15(34):4343–5.

34. Mockli GC, Silversmith M. Squamous cell carcinoma of the lung metastatic to the pancreas: diagnosis by fine-needle aspiration biopsy. Diagn Cytopathol 1997;16(3):287–8.

35. Chatzipantelis P, Salla C, Konstantinou P, et al. Endoscopic ultrasound-guided fine-needle aspiration cytology of pancreatic neuroendocrine tumors: a study of 48 cases. Cancer 2008;114(4):255–62.

36. Labate AM, Klimstra DL, Zakowski MF. Comparative cytologic features of pancreatic acinar cell carcinoma and islet cell tumor. Diagn Cytopathol 1997; 16(2):112–6.

37. Jimenez-Heffernan JA, Vicandi B, Lopez-Ferrer P, et al. Fine needle aspiration cytology of endocrine neoplasms of the pancreas. Morphologic and immunocytochemical findings in 20 cases. Acta Cytol 2004;48(3):295–301.

38. Stelow EB, Bardales RH, Shami VM, et al. Cytology of pancreatic acinar cell carcinoma. Diagn Cytopathol 2006;34(5):367–72.

39. Bardales RH, Centeno B, Mallery JS, et al. Endoscopic ultrasound-guided fine-needle aspiration cytology diagnosis of solid-pseudopapillary tumor of the pancreas: a rare neoplasm of elusive origin but characteristic cytomorphologic features. Am J Clin Pathol 2004;121(5):654–62.

40. Jani N, Dewitt J, Eloubeidi M, et al. Endoscopic ultrasound-guided fine-needle aspiration for diagnosis of solid pseudopapillary tumors of the pancreas: a multicenter experience. Endoscopy 2008;40(3):200–3.

41. Pitman MB, Faquin WC. The fine-needle aspiration biopsy cytology of pancreatoblastoma. Diagn Cytopathol 2004;31(6):402–6.

42. Zhu LC, Sidhu GS, Cassai ND, et al. Fine-needle aspiration cytology of pancreatoblastoma in a young woman: report of a case and review of the literature. Diagn Cytopathol 2005;33(4):258–62.

43. Gupta RK, Lallu S, Delahunt B. Fine-needle aspiration cytology of metastatic clear-cell renal carcinoma presenting as a solitary mass in the head of the pancreas. Diagn Cytopathol 1998;19(3):194–7.

44. Dim DC, Nugent SL, Darwin P, et al. Metastatic merkel cell carcinoma of the pancreas mimicking primary pancreatic endocrine tumor diagnosed by endoscopic ultrasound-guided fine needle aspiration cytology: a case report. Acta Cytol 2009;53(2): 223–8.

45. Adsay NV, Hasteh F, Cheng JD, et al. Lymphoepithelial cysts of the pancreas: a report of 12 cases and a review of the literature. Mod Pathol 2002;15(5): 492–501.

46. Truong LD, Stewart MG, Hao H, et al. A comprehensive characterization of lymphoepithelial cyst associated with the pancreas. Am J Surg 1995;170(1):27–32.

47. Jian B, Kimbrell HZ, Sepulveda A, et al. Lymphoepi- thelial cysts of the pancreas: endosonography- guided fine needle aspiration. Diagn Cytopathol 2008;36(9):662–5.

48. Ahlawat SK. Lymphoepithelial cyst of pancreas. Role of endoscopic ultrasound guided fine needle aspiration. JOP 2008;9(2):230–4.

49. Mandavilli SR, Port J, Ali SZ. Lymphoepithelial cyst (LEC) of the pancreas: cytomorphology and differ- ential diagnosis on fine-needle aspiration (FNA). Di- agn Cytopathol 1999;20(6):371–4.

50. Adsay NV, Hasteh F, Cheng JD, et al. Squamous- lined cysts of the pancreas: lymphoepithelial cysts, dermoid cysts (teratomas), and accessory-splenic epidermoid cysts. Semin Diagn Pathol 2000;17(1): 56–65.

51. Markovsky V, Russin VL. Fine-needle aspiration of dermoid cyst of the pancreas: a case report. Diagn Cytopathol 1993;9(1):66–9.

52. Le Borgne J, de Calan L, Partensky C. Cystadeno- mas and cystadenocarcinomas of the pancreas: a multiinstitutional retrospective study of 398 cases. French Surgical Association. Ann Surg 1999;230(2): 152–61.

53. Lal A, Bourtsos EP, DeFrias DV, et al. Microcystic adenoma of the pancreas: clinical, radiologic, and cytologic features. Cancer 2004;102(5):288–94.

54. Zamboni G, Scarpa A, Bogina G, et al. Mucinous cystic tumors of the pancreas: clinicopathological features, prognosis, and relationship to other mucinous cystic tumors. Am J Surg Pathol 1999;23(4):410–22.

55. Sole M, Iglesias C, Fernandez-Esparrach G, et al. Fine-needle aspiration cytology of intraductal papil- lary mucinous tumors of the pancreas. Cancer 2005;105(5):298–303.

56. Recine M, Kaw M, Evans DB, et al. Fine-needle aspi- ration cytology of mucinous tumors of the pancreas. Cancer 2004;102(2):92–9.

57. Stelow EB, Shami VM, Abbott TE, et al. The use of fine needle aspiration cytology for the distinction of

58. Emerson RE, Randolph ML, Cramer HM. Endo- scopic ultrasound-guided fine-needle aspiration cytology diagnosis of intraductal papillary mucinous neoplasm of the pancreas is highly predictive of pancreatic neoplasia. Diagn Cytopathol 2006; 34(7):457–62.

59. Shimizu M, Hirokawa M, Manabe T, et al. Cytologic findings in noninvasive intraductal papillary- mucinous carcinoma of the pancreas. A report of two cases. Acta Cytol 1999;43(2):243–6.

60. Brugge WR. Evaluation of pancreatic cystic lesions with EUS. Gastrointest Endosc 2004;59(6):698–707.

61. van der Waaij LA, van Dullemen HM, Porte RJ. Cyst fluid analysis in the differential diagnosis of pancre- atic cystic lesions: a pooled analysis. Gastrointest Endosc 2005;62(3):383–9.

62. Adsay NV, Merati K, Andea A, et al. The dichotomy in the preinvasive neoplasia to invasive carcinoma sequence in the pancreas: differential expression of MUC1 and MUC2 supports the existence of two separate pathways of carcinogenesis. Mod Pathol 2002;15(10):1087–95.

63. Tajiri T, Tate G, Inagaki T, et al. Intraductal tubular neoplasms of the pancreas: histogenesis and differ- entiation. Pancreas 2005;30(2):115–21.

64. Yamaguchi H, Shimizu M, Ban S, et al. Intraductal tu- bulopapillary neoplasms of the pancreas distinct from pancreatic intraepithelial neoplasia and intra- ductal papillary mucinous neoplasms. Am J Surg Pathol 2009;33(8):1164–72.

65. Klimstra DS, Adsay NV, Dhall D, et al. Intraductal tubular carcinoma of the pancreas: clinicopatho- logic and immunohistochemical analysis of 18 cases. Mod Pathol 2007;20(2):285A.

66. Chhieng DC, Benson E, Eltoum I, et al. MUC1 and MUC2 expression in pancreatic ductal carcinoma obtained by fine-needle aspiration. Cancer 2003; 99(6):365–71.

57. (continued) pancreatic mucinous neoplasia. Am J Clin Pathol 2008;129(1):67–74.

Index

Note: Page numbers of article titles are in **boldface** type.

Surgical Pathology 4 (2011) 693–697
doi:10.1016/S1875-9181(11)00109-7

surgpath.theclinics.com

Moving?

Make sure your subscription moves with you!

To notify us of your new address, find your **Clinics Account Number** (located on your mailing label above your name), and contact customer service at:

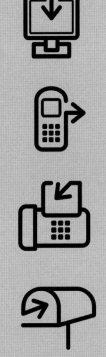

Email: journalscustomerservice-usa@elsevier.com

800-654-2452 (subscribers in the U.S. & Canada)
314-447-8871 (subscribers outside of the U.S. & Canada)

Fax number: 314-447-8029

Elsevier Health Sciences Division
Subscription Customer Service
3251 Riverport Lane
Maryland Heights, MO 63043

*To ensure uninterrupted delivery of your subscription, please notify us at least 4 weeks in advance of move.

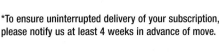